EAT RIGHT 4 YOUR TYPE

EAT RIGHT 4 YOUR TYPE

Dr Peter J. D'Adamo
with Catherine Whitney

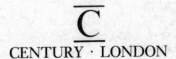

CENTURY · LONDON

This edition first published by Century Books Limited 1998 as
The Eat Right Diet

Reissued as *Eat Right 4 Your Type*, 2001

23 25 27 29 30 28 26 24 22

First published in America in 1997 as *Eat Right 4 Your Type*

Peter J. D'Adamo has asserted his right under the Copyright, Designs and
Patents Act, 1988, to be identified as the author of this work.

First published in Great Britain in 1998 by
Century

Arrow Books
Random House, 20 Vauxhall Bridge Road
London SW1V 2SA

Addresses for companies within The Random House Group
can be found at: www.randomhouse.co.uk/offices.htm

The Random House Group Limited Reg. No. 954009

A CIP catalogue record for this book is available from the British Library

ISBN 9780712677165

The Random House Group Limited supports The Forest Stewardship
Council (FSC), the leading international forest certification organisation.
All our titles that are printed on Greenpeace approved FSC certified paper
carry the FSC logo. Our paper procurement policy can be found at:
www.rbooks.co.uk/environment

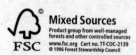

Mixed Sources
Product group from well-managed
forests and other controlled sources
www.fsc.org Cert no. TT-COC-2139
© 1996 Forest Stewardship Council

Typeset by Deltatype Ltd, Birkenhead, Merseyside
Printed and bound in Great Britain by
CPI Cox & Wyman, Reading, RG1 8EX

Contents

To the memory of my good friend,

JOHN J. MOSKO (1919–1992)

'This day is called the feast of Crispian:
He that outlives this day, and comes home safe,
Will stand a tip-toe when this day is named,
And rouse him at the name of Crispian.'

An important note

This book is not intended as a substitute for the medical recommendations of doctors or other healthcare providers. Rather, it is intended to offer information to help the reader co-operate with doctors and health professionals in a mutual quest for optimum well-being.

The identities of people described in the case histories have been changed to protect patient confidentiality.

The publisher and author are not responsible for any goods and/or services offered or referred to in this book and expressly disclaim all liability in connection with the fulfilment of orders for any such goods and/or services and for any damage, loss or expense to the person or property arising out of or relating to them.

The UK publishers have made all efforts to check that the food products recommended in this book are available in this country, and concede that some may only be found in specialist health food shops or grocers.

Acknowledgements

There are many people to thank, as no scientific pursuit is solitary. Along the way, I have been driven, inspired and supported by many people who placed their confidence in me. In particular, I give deep thanks to my wife, Martha Mosko D'Adamo, for her love and friendship; my parents, James D'Adamo Sr., N.D. and Christiana, for teaching me to trust in my intuition; and my brother, James D'Adamo Jr., for believing in me.

I am also more grateful than I can express to:

Joseph Pizzorno, N.D., for inspiring me to trust in the science of natural medicine;

Catherine Whitney, my writer, who imparted a style and organization to the raw material characteristic of a true wordsmith;

Gail Winston, the editor who long ago, out of the clear blue sky, rang me up and asked me if I wanted to write a book about natural medicine;

My literary agent, Janis Vallely, who saw the promise of my work and didn't allow it to languish somewhere in a dusty filing cabinet;

Amy Hertz, my editor at Riverhead/Putnam, whose vision turned the manuscript into the rich and important document I believe it has now become.

I am also thankful to:

Dorothy Mosko, for her invaluable assistance in the preparation of the early manuscript;

Scott Carlson, my erstwhile assistant, who never missed a UPS pickup;

Carolyn Knight, R.N., my right-hand nurse and expert phlebotomist;

Jane Dystel, Catherine's literary agent, whose advice was always on target;

Paul Krafin, who lent his sharp writing and editing skills to the revision process;

Dina Khader, R.D., who helped with the recipes and meal planning;

Michael Schacter, M.D., Jonathon Wright, M.D., and Alan Datner, M.D., for their valuable suggestions and guidance;

John Schuler, who designed the illustrations.

I also wish to thank the research interns at Bastyr University, who expertly sifted through the extensive medical literature pertaining to blood type, helping to make this book as complete an account of the subject as possible.

Lastly, I thank all the wonderful patients, who in their quest for health and happiness chose to honor me with their trust.

Introduction
The Work of Two Lives

> *I believed that no two people on the face*
> *of the earth were alike; no two people have*
> *the same fingerprints, lip prints, or*
> *voice prints. No two blades of grass or*
> *snowflakes are alike. Because I felt that*
> *all people were different from one another,*
> *I did not think it was logical that they*
> *should eat the same foods. It became clear*
> *to me that since each person was housed in*
> *a special body with different strengths,*
> *weaknesses and nutritional requirements,*
> *the only way to maintain health or cure*
> *illness was to accommodate to that*
> *particular patient's specific needs.*
>
> James D'Adamo,
> my father

Your blood type is the key that unlocks the door to the mysteries of health, disease, longevity, physical vitality and emotional strength. Your blood type determines your susceptibility to illness, which foods you should eat and how you should exercise. It is a factor in your energy levels, the efficiency with which you burn calories, your emotional response to stress and perhaps even your personality.

The connection between blood type and diet may sound radical, but it is not. We have long realized that there was a missing link in our comprehension of the process that leads either to the path of wellness or the dismal trail of disease. There had to be a reason why there were so many paradoxes in dietary studies and disease survival. There also had to be an explanation for why some people were able to lose weight on particular diets, while others were not; why some people retained vitality late into life, while others deteriorated mentally and physically. Blood type analysis has given us a way to explain these paradoxes. And the more we explore the connection, the more valid it becomes.

Blood types are as fundamental as creation itself. In the masterful logic of nature, the blood types follow an unbroken trail from the earliest moment of human creation to the present day. They are the signature of our ancient ancestors on the indestructible parchment of history.

Now we have begun to discover how to use the blood type as a cellular fingerprint that unravels many of the major mysteries surrounding our quest for good health. This work is an extension of the recent groundbreaking findings concerning human DNA. Our understanding of blood type takes the science of genetics one step further by stating unequivocally that every human being is utterly unique. There is no right or wrong lifestyle or diet; there are only right or wrong choices to be made based on our individual genetic codes.

How I Found the Missing Blood Type Link

My work in the field of blood type analysis is the fulfilment of a lifetime pursuit – not only my own but also my father's. I am a second-generation naturopathic physician. Dr James D'Adamo, my father, graduated from naturopathic college (a four-year postgraduate programme) in 1957 and later studied in Europe at several of the great spas. He noticed that although many patients did well on strict vegetarian and low-fat diets, which are the hallmarks of 'spa cuisine', a certain number of patients did not appear to improve, and some did poorly or even worsened. A sensitive man with keen powers of deduction and insight, my father reasoned that there should be some sort of blueprint that he could use to determine differences in the dietary needs of his patients. He rationalized that since blood was the fundamental source of nourishment to the body, perhaps some aspect of the blood could help to identify these differences. My father set about testing this theory by blood typing his patients and observing individualized reactions when they were prescribed different diets.

Through the years and with countless patients, a pattern began to emerge. He noticed that patients who were Type A seemed to do poorly on high-protein diets that included generous portions of meat, but did very well on vegetable proteins such as soya and tofus. Dairy products tended to produce copious amounts of mucus discharge in the sinuses and respiratory passages of Type As. When told to increase their levels of physical activity and exercise, Type As usually felt fatigued and unwell; when they performed lighter forms of exercise, such as yoga, they felt alert and energized.

On the other hand, Type O patients thrived on high-protein diets, and they felt invigorated by intense physical activities, such as jogging and aerobics. The more my father tested the different blood types, the greater his conviction became that each of them followed a distinct path to wellness.

Inspired by the saying 'One man's food is another man's poison', my father condensed his observations and dietary recommendations into a book he titled *One Man's Food*. When the book was published in 1980, I was in my third year of naturopathic studies at Seattle's John Bastyr College. During this time revolutionary gains were being achieved in naturopathic education. The goal of Bastyr College was nothing less than to produce the complete alternative physician, the intellectual and scientific equal of a medical internist, but with specialized naturopathic training. For the first time naturopathic techniques, procedures and substances could be scientifically evaluated with the benefits of modern technology. I waited for an opportunity to research my father's blood type theory. I wanted to assure myself that it carried valid scientific weight.

My chance came in 1982 when, for a clinical rounds requirement in my senior year, I began scanning the medical literature to see if I could find any correlation between the ABO blood types and a predilection for certain diseases, and whether any of this supported my father's diet theory. Since my father's book was based on his subjective impressions of the blood types rather than on an objective method of evaluation, I wasn't certain that I would be able to find any scientific basis for his theories. But I was amazed at what I learned.

My first breakthrough came with the discovery that two major diseases of the stomach were associated with blood type. The first was the peptic ulcer, a condition often related to higher than average stomach acid levels. This condition was reported to be more common in people with Type O blood than in people with other blood types. I was immediately intrigued, since my father had observed that Type O patients did well on animal products and protein diets – foods that require more stomach acid for proper digestion.

The second correlation was an association between Type A and stomach cancer. Stomach cancer was often linked to low levels of stomach acid production, as was pernicious anaemia, another disorder found more often in Type A individuals. Pernicious anaemia is related to a lack of vitamin B12, which requires sufficient stomach acid for its absorption.

As I studied these facts I realized that on the one hand, Type O blood predisposed people to an illness associated with too much stomach acid, while on the other hand, Type A blood predisposed people to two illnesses associated with too little stomach acid. That was the link I'd been looking for. There was absolutely a scientific basis for my father's observations. And so began my ongoing love affair with the science and anthropology of the blood types. In time, I found that my father's initial work on the correlation between blood type, diet and health was far more significant than he had ever imagined.

Four Simple Keys to Unlock Life's Mysteries

I grew up in a family that was mostly Blood Type A, and because of my father's work we ate a basically vegetarian diet consisting of foods such as tofu, steamed vegetables and salads. As a child I was often embarrassed and felt somewhat deprived, because none of my friends ate weird foods like tofu. On the contrary, they were happily engaged in another kind of 'diet revolution' sweeping America in the 1950s; their diets consisted of hamburgers, hot dogs, greasy chips, candy bars, ice-cream and lots of fizzy drinks.

Today, I still eat the way I did as a child, and I love it. Every day I eat the foods that my Type A body craves, and it's immensely satisfying.

In *Eat Right 4 Your Type* I will teach you about the fundamental relationship between your blood type and the dietary and lifestyle choices that will help you live at your very best. The essence of the blood type connection rests in these facts:

- Your blood type – O, A, B or AB – is a powerful genetic fingerprint that identifies you as surely as your DNA.
- When you use the individualized characteristics of your blood type as a guide for eating and living you will be healthier, you will easily reach your ideal weight and you will slow the process of ageing.
- Your blood type is a more reliable measure of your identity than race, culture or geography. It is a genetic blueprint for who you are, a guide to how you can live most fully.
- The key to the significance of blood type can be found in the story of human evolution: Type O is the oldest; Type A evolved with the agrarian society; Type B emerged as humans migrated north into colder, harsher territories; and Type AB was a thoroughly modern adaptation, a result of the intermingling of disparate groups. This evolutionary story relates directly to the dietary needs of each blood type today.

What is this remarkable factor, the blood type?

Blood type is one of several medically recognized variations, much like hair and eye colour. Many of these variations, such as fingerprint patterns and the more recent DNA analysis, are used extensively by forensic scientists and criminologists, as well as those who research the causes and cures of disease. Blood type is every bit as significant as other variations; in many ways, it's a more useful measure. Blood type analysis is a logical system. The information is simple to learn and easy to follow. I've taught the system to numerous doctors, who tell me they are getting good results with patients who are following its guidelines. Now I will teach it to you. By learning the principles of blood type analysis, you can tailor the optimal diet for yourself and your family members. You can pinpoint the foods that make you sick, contribute to weight gain and lead to chronic disease.

Early on, I realized that blood type analysis offered a powerful means of interpreting individual variations in health and disease. Given the amount of available research data, it is surprising that the effects of blood type on our health have not received the measure of attention that they deserve. But now I am prepared to make that information available – not just to my fellow scientists and colleagues in the medical community, but to you.

At first glance, the science of blood type may seem daunting, but I assure you it is as simple and basic as life itself. I will tell you about the ancient trail of the evolution of blood types (as riveting as the story of human history), and demystify the science of blood types to provide a clear and simple plan that you will be able to follow.

Maybe this all sounds a little to obvious to you. Maybe this sounds a little far-fetched. But even if you don't believe it will work, just try it for two weeks. Stick to the letter of your blood type diet for just two weeks. My patients have experienced increased energy and the beginnings of weight loss after that short period of time. Give your blood type diet a chance to bring you the benefits I've seen it bring to the more than 4000 people I've put on the diet. Blood not only provides our most vital nourishment, but now proves itself a vehicle for our future well-being.

Peter D'Adamo
June 1996

PART ONE

YOUR BLOOD TYPE IDENTITY

1
Blood Type: The Real Evolution Revolution

BLOOD IS LIFE itself. It is the primal force which fuels the power and mystery of birth, the horrors of disease, war and violent death. Entire civilizations have been built on blood ties. Tribes, clans and monarchies depend on them. We cannot exist without blood – literally or figuratively.

Blood is magical. Blood is mystical. Blood is alchemical. It appears throughout human history as a profound religious and cultural symbol. Ancient peoples mixed it together and drank it to denote unity and fealty. From the earliest times, hunters performed rituals to appease the spirits of the animals they killed by offering up the animal blood and smearing it on their faces and bodies. The blood of the lamb was placed as a mark on the hovels of the slave Jews of Egypt so that the Angel of Death would pass over them. Moses is said to have turned the waters of Egypt to blood in his quest to free his people. The symbolic blood of Jesus Christ has been, for nearly 2000 years, central to the most sacred rite of Christianity.

Blood evokes such rich and sacred imagery because it is in reality so extraordinary. Not only does it supply the complex delivery and defence systems that are necessary for our very existence, it provides a keystone for humanity – a looking-glass through which we can trace the faint tracks of our journey.

In the last forty years we have been able to use biological markers such as blood type to map the movements and groupings of our ancestors. By learning how these early people adapted to the challenges posed by constantly changing climates, germs and diets, we are learning about ourselves. Change in climate and available food produced new blood types. Blood type is the unbroken cord that binds us.

Ultimately, the differences in blood types reflect upon the human ability to acclimatize to different environmental challenges. For the most part, these challenges impacted the digestive and immune systems: a piece of bad meat could kill you; a cut or scrape could evolve into a deadly infection. Yet the human race survived. And the story of that survival is inextricably tied to our digestive and immune systems. It is in these two areas that most of the distinctions between blood types are found.

THE HUMAN STORY

The story of humankind is the story of survival. More specifically, it is the story of where humans lived and what they could eat there. It is about food – finding food and moving to find food. We don't know for certain when human evolution began. Neanderthals, the first humanoids we can recognize, may have developed 500,000 years ago – or maybe even earlier. We do know human prehistory began in Africa, where we evolved from human-like creatures. Early life was short, nasty and brutish. People died a thousand different ways – opportunistic infections, parasites, animal attacks, broken bones, childbirth – and they died young.

Neanderthals probably ate a rather crude diet of wild plants, grubs and the scavenged leftovers from the kills of predatory animals. They were more prey than predator, especially when it came to infections and parasitic afflictions. (Many of the parasites, worms, flukes and infectious micro-organisms found in Africa do not stimulate the immune system to produce a specific antibody to them, probably because the early Type O people already had protection in the form of the antibodies they carried from birth.)

As the human race moved around and was forced to adapt its diet to changing conditions, the new diet provoked adaptations in the digestive tract and immune system necessary for it to first survive and later thrive in each new habitat. These changes are reflected in the development of the blood types, which appear to have arrived at critical junctures of human development:

1. The ascent of humans to the top of the food chain (evolution of **Type O** to its fullest expression).
2. The change from hunter-gatherer to a more domesticated agrarian lifestyle (appearance of **Type A**).
3. The merging and migration of the races from the African homeland to Europe, Asia and the Americas (development of **Type B**).
4. The modern intermingling of disparate groups (the arrival of **Type AB**).

Each blood type contains the genetic message of our ancestors' diets and behaviours and although we're a long way away from early history, many of their traits still affect us. Knowing these predispositions helps us to understand the logic of the blood type diets.

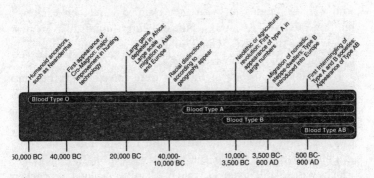

The blood type–anthropology timeline. Starting from earliest times, the diagram highlights various human developments in relation to the introduction of the blood types. Interestingly, the evolutionary changes in blood type have almost a biblical time frame. When everyone was Type O (the longest period of time), and they occupied a contracted living space, ate the same diet, and breathed in the same organisms, any further change was unnecessary. However, with the increase in population and subsequent migrations, variation accelerated. The subsequent Blood Types A and B are no more than 15,000 to 25,000 years old, and Type AB is far more recent.

O is for Old

The appearance of our Cro-Magnon ancestors around 40,000 BC propelled the human species to the top of the food chain, making them the most dangerous predators on earth. They began to hunt in organized packs; in a short time, they were able to make weapons and use tools. These major advances gave them strength and superiority beyond their natural physical abilities.

Skilful and formidable hunters, the Cro-Magnons soon had little to fear from any of their animal rivals. With no natural predators other than themselves, the population exploded. Protein (meat) was their fuel, and it was at this point that the digestive attributes of Blood Type O reached their fullest expression.

Humans thrived on meat, and it took a remarkably short time for them to kill off the big game within their hunting range. There were more and more people to feed, so competition for meat became intense. Hunters began fighting and killing others who were impinging on what they claimed were their exclusive hunting grounds. As always, human beings found their greatest enemy to be themselves. Good hunting areas became scarce. The migration of the human race began.

By 30,000 BC, bands of hunters were travelling further and further in search of meat. When a shift in the trade winds desiccated what had been fertile hunting land in the African Sahara, and when previously frozen northern areas grew warmer, they began to move out of Africa into Europe and Asia.

This movement seeded the planet with its base population, which was Blood Type O, the predominant blood type even today.

By 20,000 BC Cro-Magnons had moved fully into Europe and Asia, decimating the vast herds of large game to such an extent that other foods had to be found. Searching each new area for anything edible, it is likely that the carnivorous humans quickly became omnivorous, with a mixed diet of berries, grubs, nuts, roots and small animals. Populations also thrived along the coastlines and the teeming lakes and rivers of the earth where fish and other food was abundant. By 10,000 BC, humans occupied every main land mass on the planet, except Antarctica.

The movement of the early humans to less temperate climates created lighter skins, less massive bone structures and straighter

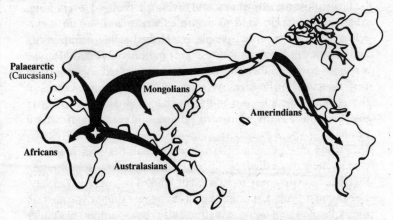

From their base in the ancestral homeland of Africa, early Blood Type O hunter-gatherers wandered throughout Africa and into Europe and Asia in search of new supplies of large game. As they encountered changing environmental conditions, they began to develop modern racial characteristics.

---

hair. Nature, over time, re-acclimatized them to the regions of the earth they inhabited. People moved northwards, so light skin developed, which was better protected against frostbite than dark skin. Lighter skin was also better able to metabolize vitamin D in a land of shorter days and longer nights.

The Cro-Magnons eventually burned themselves out; their success was anathema. Overpopulation soon exhausted the available hunting grounds. What had once seemed like an unending supply of large game animals diminished sharply. This led to increased competition for the remaining meat. Competition led to war, and war to further migration.

A is for Agrarian
Type A blood initially appeared somewhere in Asia or the Middle East between 25,000 and 15,000 BC in response to new environmental conditions. It emerged at the peak of the Neolithic Period, or New Stone Age, which followed the Old Stone Age, or Paleolithic period, of the Cro-Magnon hunters. Agriculture and animal domestication were the hallmarks of its culture.

The cultivation of grains and livestock changed everything. Able to forgo their hand-to-mouth existence and sustain themselves for the first time, people established stable communities and permanent living structures. This radically different lifestyle, a major change in diet and environment, resulted in an entirely new mutation in the digestive tracts and the immune systems of the Neolithic peoples – a mutation that allowed them to better tolerate and absorb cultivated grains and other agricultural products. Type A was born.

Settling into permanent farming communities presented new developmental challenges. The skills necessary for hunting together now gave way to a different kind of co-operative society. For the first time, a specific skill at doing one thing depended on the skills of others doing something else. For example, the miller was dependent on the farmer to bring in his crops; the farmer depended upon the miller to grind his grain. One no longer thought of food as only an immediate source of nourishment or as a sometime thing. Fields needed to be sown and cultivated in anticipation of future reward. Planning and networking with others became the order of the day. Psychologically, these are traits at which Type As excel – perhaps another environmental adaptation.

The gene for Type A began to thrive in the early agrarian societies. The genetic mutation that produced Type A from Type O occurred rapidly – so rapidly that the rate of mutation was comparable to four times that of *Drasophila*, the common fruitfly and current record holder!

What could have been the reason for this extraordinary rate of human mutation from Type O to Type A? It was survival. Survival of the fittest in a crowded society. Because Type A emerged as more resistant to infections common to densely populated areas, urban, industrialized societies quickly became Type A. Even today, survivors of plague, cholera and smallpox show a predominance of Type A over Type O.

Eventually the gene for Type A blood spread beyond Asia and the Middle East into western Europe, carried by the Indo-Europeans, who penetrated deeply into the pre-Neolithic populations. The Indo-European hordes appeared originally in south central Russia, and between 2500 and 2000 BC pushed southwards into the top of south-western Asia, creating the populations and peoples of Iran and Afghanistan. Ever burgeoning, they moved further westwards into Europe.

The Indo-European invasion was really the original diet revolution. It introduced new foods and lifestyle habits into the simpler immune systems and digestive tracts of the early hunter-gatherers, and those changes were so profound that they produced the environmental stress necessary to spread the type A gene. In time, the digestive system of the hunter-gatherers lost its ability to digest its carnivorous pre-agricultural diet.

Today, Type A blood is still found in its highest concentration among western Europeans. The frequency of Type A diminishes as we head eastwards from western Europe, following the receding trails of the ancient migratory patterns. Type A peoples are highly concentrated across the Mediterranean, Adriatic and Aegean seas, particularly in Corsica, Sardinia, Spain, Turkey and the Balkans. The Japanese also have some of the highest concentrations of Type As in eastern Asia, along with a moderately high number of Blood Type Bs.

Blood Type A had mutated from Type O in response to the myriad infections provoked by an increased populace and major dietary changes. But Blood Type B was different.

B is for Balance

Blood Type B developed sometime between 10,000 and 15,000 BC, in the area of the Himalayan highlands – now part of Pakistan and India.

Pushed from the hot, lush savannahs of eastern Africa to the cold, unyielding highlands of the Himalayas, Blood Type B may have initially mutated in response to climactic changes. It first appeared in India or the Ural region of Asia among a mix of Caucasian and Mongolian tribes. This new blood type was soon characteristic of the great tribes of steppe dwellers, who by this time dominated the Eurasian plains.

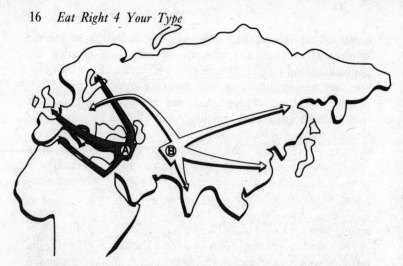

Origins and movements of Type A and Type B. From its beginnings in Asia and the Middle East, the gene for Type A was carried by Indo-European peoples into western and northern Europe. Other migrations carried Type A into northern Africa, where it spread into the Saharan Africans. From its origins in the western Himalayan mountains, Type B was carried by Mongolian peoples into southeast Asia and into the Asian flatlands or steppes. A separate migration of Type B peoples entered eastern Europe. By this time the sea levels of the earth had risen, removing the land bridge between North America and Asia. This prevented any movement of Type B into North America, where the earlier populations continued on as exclusively Type O.

As the Mongolians swept through Asia, the gene for Type B blood was firmly entrenched. The Mongolians spread northwards pursuing a culture dependent upon herding and domesticating animals – as their diet of meat and cultured dairy products reflected.

Two distinct Type Bs sprang up as the pastoral nomads pushed into Asia: an agrarian, comparatively sedentary group in the south and the east; and a nomadic, war-like society conquering the north and the west. The nomads were expert horsemen who penetrated far into eastern Europe, and the gene for Type B blood is still in strong evidence in many of the eastern European populations. In the meantime, an entire agriculturally based culture had spread throughout China and south-east Asia. Because of the nature of the land they chose to till, and climates unique to their areas, these peoples created and employed sophisticated irrigation and cultivation techniques that displayed an awesome blend of creativity, intelligence and engineering.

The schism between the warlike tribes to the north and the peaceful farmers to the south was deep, and its remnants exist to this day in Southern Asian cuisine, which uses little if any dairy foods. To the Asian mind, dairy products are the food of the barbarian, which is unfortunate because the diet they have adopted does not suit Type Bs as well.

Of all the ABO types, Type B shows the most clearly defined geographic distribution. Stretching as a great belt across the Eurasian plains and down to the Indian subcontinent, Type B is found in increased numbers from Japan, Mongolia, China, and India up to the Ural Mountains. From there westward, the percentages fall until a low is reached at the western tip of Europe.

The small numbers of Type B in old and western Europeans represents western migration by Asian nomadic peoples. This is best seen in the easternmost western Europeans, the Germans and Austrians, who have an unexpectedly high incidence of Type B blood compared to their western neighbours. The highest occurrence of Type B in Germans occurs in the area around the upper and middle Elbe river, which had been nominally held as the dividing line between civilization and barbarism in ancient times.

Modern sub-continental Indians, a Caucasian people, have some of the highest frequencies of Type B blood in the world. The northern Chinese and Koreans have very high rates of Type B blood and very low rates of Type A.

The blood type characteristics of the various Jewish populations have long been of interest to anthropologists. As a general rule, regardless of their nationality or race, there is a trend towards higher than average rates of Type B blood. The Ashkenazim and the Sephardim, the two major Jewish sects, share strong levels of Type B blood, and appear to have very few differences. The pre-Diaspora Babylonian Jews differ considerably from the primarily Type O Arabic population of Iraq (the location of the biblical Babylon) in that they are primarily Type B, with some frequency of Type A.

AB is for Modern

Type AB blood is rare. Emerging from the intermingling of Type A Caucasians with Type B Mongolians, it is found in less than 5 per cent of the population, and it is the newest of the blood types.

Until ten or twelve centuries ago, there was no Type AB blood. Attila the Hun and other barbarian hordes sliced through the soft underbelly of any collapsing civilizations, overrunning the length and breadth of the Roman Empire. As a result of the intermingling of these Eastern invaders with the last trembling vestiges of European civilization, Type AB blood came into being. No evidence for the occurrence of this blood type extends beyond 900–1000 years ago, when a large western migration of eastern peoples took place. Blood Type AB is rarely found in European graves prior to AD 900. Studies on prehistoric grave exhumations in Hungary show a distinct lack of this blood group into the Langobard age (4th to 7th century AD). This would seem to indicate that up until that point in time, European populations of Type A and Type B did not come into common contact, or if so, did not mingle or intermarry.

Because Type ABs inherit the tolerance of both Type A and Type B, their immune systems have an enhanced ability to manufacture more specific antibodies to microbial infections. This unique quality of possessing neither anti-A or anti-B antibodies minimizes their chances of being prone to allergies and other autoimmune diseases like arthritis, inflammation and lupus. There is, however, a greater predisposition to certain cancers because Type AB responds to anything A-like or B-like as 'self', so it manufactures no opposing antibodies.

Type AB presents a multi-faceted, and sometimes perplexing, blood type identity. It is the first blood type to adopt an amalgamation of immune characteristics, some of which make them stronger, and some of which are in conflict. Perhaps Type AB presents the perfect metaphor for modern life: complex and unsettled.

The Blending Grounds

Blood type, geography and race are woven together to form our human identity. We may have cultural differences, but when you look at blood type, you see how superficial they are. Your blood type is older than your race and more fundamental than your ethnicity. The blood types were not a hit or miss act of random genetic activity. Each new blood type was an evolutionary response to a series of cataclysmic chain reactions, spread over aeons of environmental upheaval and change.

Although the early racial changes seem to have occurred in a world that was composed almost exclusively of Type O blood, the racial diversifications, coupled with dietary, environmental and geographical adaptations, were part of the evolutionary engine that ultimately produced the other blood types.

Some anthropologists believe that classifying humans into races invites over-simplification. Blood type is a far more important determinant of individuality and similarity than race. For example, an African and Caucasian of Type A blood could exchange blood or organs and have many of the same aptitudes, digestive functions and immunological structures – characteristics they would not share with a member of their own race who was Blood Type B.

Racial distinctions based on skin colours, ethnic practices, geographical homelands or cultural roots are not a valid way to distinguish peoples. Mankind has a lot more in common with one another than we may have ever suspected. We are all potentially brothers and sisters – in blood.

* * *

Today, as we look back on this remarkable evolutionary revolution, it is clear that our ancestors had unique biological blueprints that complemented their environments. It is this lesson we bring with us into our current understanding of blood types, for the genetic characteristics of our ancestors live in our blood today.

- **Type O**
  The oldest and most basic blood type, the survivor at the top of the food chain, with a strong and ornery immune system willing to and capable of destroying anyone, friend or foe.
- **Type A**
  The first immigrants, forced by the necessity of migration to adapt to a more agrarian diet and lifestyle – and a more co-operative personality to get along in crowded communities.
- **Type B**
  The assimilator, adapting to new climates and the mingling of populations; representing nature's quest for a more balanced force between the tensions of the mind and the demands of the immune system.
- **Type AB**
  The delicate offspring of a rare merger between the tolerant Type A and the formerly barbaric but more balanced Type B.

Our ancestors left each of us a special legacy, imprinted in our blood types. This legacy exists permanently in the nucleus of each cell. It is here that the anthropology and science of our blood meet.

2
Blood Code: The Blueprint of Blood Type

BLOOD IS A force of nature, the *élan vital* that has sustained us since time immemorial. A single drop of blood, too small to see with the naked eye, contains the entire genetic code of a human being. The DNA blueprint is intact and replicated within us endlessly – through our blood.

Our blood also contains aeons of genetic memory – bits and pieces of specific programming, passed on from our ancestors in codes we are still attempting to comprehend. One such code rests within our blood type. Perhaps it is the most important code we can decipher in our attempt to unravel the mysteries of blood and its vital role in our existence.

To the naked eye, blood is a homogenous red liquid. But under the microscope blood shows itself to be composed of many different elements. The abundant red blood cells contain a special type of iron that our bodies use to carry oxygen and create the blood's characteristic rust colour. White blood cells, far less numerous than red, cruise our bloodstreams like ever-vigilant troops, protecting us against infection.

This complex, living fluid also contains proteins that deliver nutrients to the tissues, platelets that help it to clot and plasma that contains the guardians of our immune system.

The Importance of Blood Type
You may be unaware of your own blood type unless you've donated blood or needed a transfusion. Most people think of blood type as an inert factor, something that only comes into play when there is a hospital emergency. But now that you have heard

the dramatic story of the evolution of blood type, you are beginning to understand that blood type has always been the driving force behind human survival, changing and adapting to new conditions, environments and foods supplies.

Why is our blood type so powerful? What is the essential role it plays in our survival – not just thousands of years ago, but today?

Your blood type is the key to your body's entire immune system. It controls the influence of viruses, bacteria, infections, chemicals, stress and the entire assortment of invaders and conditions that might compromise your immune system.

The word 'immune' comes from the Latin *immunis*, which denoted a city in the Roman Empire that was not required to pay taxes. (If only your blood type could give you that kind of immunity!) The immune system works to define 'self' and destroy 'non-self'. This is a critical function, for without it your immune system could attack your own tissues by mistake or allow a dangerous organism access to vital areas of your body. In spite of all its complexity, the immune system boils down to two basic functions: recognizing 'us' and killing 'them'. In this respect your body is like a large invitation-only party. If the prospective guest supplies the correct invitation, the security guards allow him to enter and enjoy himself. If an invitation is lacking or forged, the guest is forcefully removed.

Enter the Blood Type

Nature has endowed our immune systems with very sophisticated methods to determine if a substance in the body is foreign or not. One method involves chemical markers called *antigens* which are found on the cells of our bodies. Every life form, from the simplest virus to humans themselves, has unique antigens that form a part of their chemical fingerprint. One of the most powerful antigens in the human body is the one that determines your blood type. The different blood type antigens are so sensitive that when they are operating effectively, they are the immune system's greatest security system. When your immune system sizes up a suspicious character (i.e. a foreign antigen from bacteria) one of the first things it looks for is your blood type antigen to tell it whether the intruder is friend or foe.

Each blood type possesses a different antigen with its own special chemical structure. Your blood type is named for the blood type antigen you possess on your red blood cells.

IF YOU ARE	ANTIGEN(S) ON YOUR CELLS
Blood Type A	A
Blood Type B	B
Blood Type AB	A and B
Blood Type O	no antigens

Visualize the chemical structure of blood types as antennae of sorts, projecting outwards from the surface of our cells into deep space. These antennae are made from long chains of a repeating sugar called fucose, which by itself forms the simplest of the blood types, the O antigen of Blood Type O. The early discoveries of blood type called it 'O' as a way to make us think of 'zero' or 'no real antigen'. This antenna also serves as the base for the other Blood Types, A, B and AB.

- **Blood Type A** is formed when the O antigen, or fucose, plus another sugar called N-acetyl-galactosamine, is added. So, fucose plus N-acetyl-galactosamine equals Blood Type A.
- **Blood Type B** is also based on the O antigen, or fucose, but has a different sugar, named D-galactosamine, added on. So, fucose plus D-galactosamine equals Blood Type B.
- **Blood Type AB** is based on the O antigen, fucose, plus the two sugars, N-acetyl-galactosamine and D-galactosamine. So, fucose plus N-acetyl-galactosamine plus D-galactosamine equals Blood Type AB.

At this point you may be wondering about other blood type identifiers, like positive and negative, or secretor/non-secretor. Usually, when people state their blood types they say, 'I'm A positive' or, 'I'm O negative'. These variations, or sub-groups,

The Four Blood Types And Their Antigens

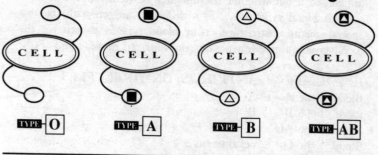

key -

⬭ CELL

◖ Fucose > basic sugar

■ N-acetyl-galactosamine > A sugar

△ D-galactosamine > B sugar

◣ N-acetyl-galactosamine + D-glactosamine > AB sugar

The four blood types and their antigens. Type O is the stalk, fucose; Type A is fucose plus the sugar N-acetyl-galactosamine; Type B is fucose plus the sugar D-galactosamine; Type AB is fucose plus the A-sugar and the B-sugar.

within blood types play relatively insignificant roles. More than 90 per cent of all the factors associated with your blood type are related to your primary type – O, A, B, or AB. (See Appendix E for details on the meaning of the subgroups.) We will concentrate on your blood type itself.

Antigens Create Antibodies (Immune System Smart Bombs)

When your blood type antigen senses that a foreign antigen has entered the system, the first thing it does is create antibodies to that antigen. These antibodies, specialized chemicals manufactured by the cells of the immune system, are designed to attach to and tag the foreign antigen for destruction.

Antibodies are the cellular equivalent of the military's smart bomb. The cells of our immune system manufacture countless varieties of antibodies, and each is specifically designed to identify and attach to one particular foreign antigen. A continual battle wages between the immune system and intruders who try to change or mutate their antigens into some new form that the body will not recognize. The immune system responds to this challenge with an ever-increasing inventory of antibodies.

When an antibody encounters the antigen of a microbial interloper, a reaction called agglutination (gluing) occurs. The antibody attaches itself to the viral antigen and makes it very sticky. When cells, viruses, parasites and bacteria are agglutinated, they stick together and clump up, which makes the job of their disposal all the easier. As microbes must rely on their slippery powers of evasion, this is a very powerful defence mechanism. It is rather like handcuffing criminals together; they become far less dangerous than when they are allowed to move around freely. Sweeping the system of odd cells, viruses, parasites and bacteria, the antibodies herd the undesirables together for easy identification and disposal.

The system of blood type antigens and antibodies has other ramifications besides detecting microbial and other invaders. Nearly a century ago, Dr Karl Landsteiner, a brilliant Austrian physician and scientist, also found that blood types produced antibodies to other blood types. His revolutionary discovery explained why some people could exchange blood, while others could not. Until Dr Landsteiner's time, blood transfusions were a hit and miss affair. Sometimes they 'took', and sometimes they didn't and nobody knew why. Thanks to Dr Landsteiner, we now know which blood types are recognized as friend by other blood types, and which are recognized as foe.

Dr. Landsteiner learned that:

- Blood Type A carried anti-B antibodies. Type B would be rejected by Type A.
- Blood Type B carried anti-A antibodies. Type A would be rejected by Type B.

Thus, Type A and Type B could not exchange blood.

- Blood Type AB carried no antibodies. The universal receiver, it would accept any other blood type! But, because it carried both A and B antigens, it would be rejected by all other blood types.

Thus, Type AB could receive blood from everyone, but could give blood to no one (except another Type AB, of course).

• Blood Type O carried anti-A and anti-B antibodies. Type A, Type B and Type AB would be rejected.

Thus, Type O could not receive blood from anyone but another Type O. But, free of A-like and B-like antigens, Type O could give blood to everyone else. Type O is the universal donor!

IF YOU ARE	YOU CARRY ANTIBODIES AGAINST
Blood Type A	Blood Type B
Blood Type B	Blood Type A
Blood Type AB	No antibodies
Blood Type O	Blood Type A and B

The 'anti-other-blood-type' antibodies are the strongest antibodies in our immune system, and their ability to clump (agglutinate) the blood cells of an opposing blood type is so powerful that it can be immediately observed on a glass slide with the unaided eye. Most of our other antibodies require some sort of stimulation (such as a vaccination or an infection) for their production. The blood type antibodies are different: they are produced automatically, often appearing at birth and reaching almost adult levels by four months of age.

But there is much more to the agglutination story. It was also found that many foods agglutinate the cells of certain blood types (in a way similar to rejection) but not others, meaning that a food which may be harmful to the cells of one blood type may be beneficial to the cells of another. Not surprisingly, many of the antigens in these foods had A-like or B-like characteristics. This discovery provided the scientific link between blood type and diet. Remarkably, however, its revolutionary implications would lie dormant, gathering dust for most of this century – until a handful of scientists, doctors and nutritionists began to explore the connection.

Lectins: The Diet Connection

A chemical reaction occurs between your blood and the foods that you eat. This reaction is part of your genetic inheritance. It is amazing but true that today, in the late twentieth century, your immune and digestive systems still maintain a favouritism for foods that your blood type ancestors ate.

We know this because of a factor called lectins. Lectins, abundant and diverse proteins found in foods, have agglutinating properties that affect your blood. Lectins are a powerful way for organisms to attach themselves to other organisms in nature. Lots of germs, and even our own immune systems, used this super-glue to their benefit. For example, cells in our liver's bile ducts have lectins on their surfaces to help them snatch up bacteria and parasites. Bacteria and other microbes have lectins on their surfaces, as well, which work rather like suction cups, so they can attach to the slippery mucousal linings of the body. Often, the lectins used by viruses or bacteria can be blood type specific, making them a stickier pest for a person of that blood type.

So, too, with the lectins in food. When you eat a food containing protein lectins that are incompatible with your blood type antigen, the lectins target an organ or bodily system (kidney, liver, brain, stomach, etc.) and begin to agglutinate blood cells in that area.

Many food lectins have characteristics that are close enough to a certain blood type antigen to make it an 'enemy' to another. For example, milk has B-like qualities; if a person with Type A blood drinks it, their system will immediately start the agglutination process in order to reject it.

Here's an example of how a lectin agglutinates in the body. Let's say a Type A person drinks a glass of milk. The milk is digested in the stomach through the process of acid hydrolysis. However, the lectin protein is resistant to acid hydrolysis. It doesn't get digested, but stays intact. It may interact directly with the lining of the stomach or intestinal tract, or it may get absorbed into our bloodstream along with the digested milk nutrients. Different lectins target different organs and body systems.

Once the intact lectin protein settles somewhere in your body, it literally has a magnetic effect on the cells in that region. It clumps the cells together and they are targeted for destruction, as if they, too, were foreign invaders. This clumping can cause irritable bowel syndrome in the intestines, cirrhosis of the liver, or block the flow of blood through the kidneys – to name just a few of the effects.

Lectins: A Dangerous Glue

You may remember the bizarre assassination of Gyorgi Markov in 1978 on a London street. Markov was killed by an unknown Soviet KGB agent while waiting for a bus. Initially, the autopsy could not pinpoint how it was done. After a thorough search, however, a tiny gold bead was found embedded in Markov's leg. The bead was found to be permeated with a chemical called ricin, which is a toxic lectin extracted from castor beans. Ricin is so potent an agglutinin that even an infinitesimally small amount can cause death by swiftly converting the body's red blood cells into large clots which block the arteries. Ricin kills instantaneously.

Fortunately, most lectins found in the diet are not quite so life-theatening, although they can cause a variety of other problems, especially if they are specific to a particular blood type. For the most part our immune systems protect us from lectins. Ninety-five per cent of the lectins we absorb from our typical diets are sloughed off by the body. But at least 5 per cent of the lectins we eat are filtered into the blood stream, where they react with and destroy red and white blood cells. The actions of lectins in the digestive tract can be even more powerful. There, they often create a violent inflammation of the sensitive mucus of the intestines, and this agglutinative action may mimic food allergies. Even a minute quantity of a lectin is capable of agglutinating a huge number of cells if the particular blood type is reactive.

This is not to say that you should suddenly become fearful of every food you eat. After all, lectins are widely abundant in pulses, seafood, grains and vegetables. It's hard to bypass them. The key is to avoid the lectins that agglutinate your particular cells – determined by blood type. For example, gluten, the most common lectin found in wheat and other grains, binds to the lining of the small intestine, causing substantial inflammation and painful irritation in some blood types – especially Type O.

Lectins vary widely according to their source. For example, the lectin found in wheat has a different shape and attaches to a different combination of sugars than the lectin found in soya, making each of these foods dangerous for some blood types, but beneficial for others.

Nervous tissue as a rule is very sensitive to the agglutinating effect of food lectins. This may explain why some researchers feel that allergy-avoidance diets may be of benefit in treating certain types of nervous disorders, such as hyperactivity. Russian researchers have noted that the brains of schizophrenics are more sensitive to the attachment of certain common food lectins.

Injections of lentil lectin into the knee-joint cavities of non-sensitized rabbits resulted in the development of arthritis that was indistinguishable from rheumatoid arthritis. Many people with arthritis feel that avoiding the so-called 'nightshade' vegetables, such as tomatoes, aubergines and white potatoes, seems to help their arthritis. That's not surprising, since most nightshades are very high in lectins.

Food lectins can also interact with the surface receptors of the body's white cells, programming them to multiply rapidly. These lectins are called mitogens because they cause the white cells to enter mitosis, the process of cell reproduction. They do not clump blood by gluing cells together; they merely attach themselves to things, like fleas on a dog. Occasionally an emergency room doctor will be faced with a very ill but otherwise aparently normal child who has an extraordinarily high white blood cell count. Although paediatric leukaemia is usually the first thing to come to mind, the astute doctor will ask the parent, 'Was your child playing in the garden?' If the answer is yes, 'Was he eating any weeds or putting plants in his mouth?' It may turn out that the child was eating the leaves or shoots of the

Blood Type–Specific Food Lectins

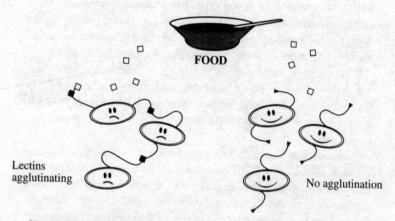

FOOD

Lectins
agglutinating

No agglutination

Since each blood type antigen possesses a unique shape, many lectins interact with one specific blood type because they fit the shape of that particular blood type. In the example above, food lectins from a steaming plate of lima beans interact and agglutinate Type A cells (on the left) because they fit the shape of the A antigen. The antigen for Type B blood (on the right), a different sugar molecule with a different shape, is not affected. Conversely, a food lectin (such as buckwheat) that can specifically attach to and agglutinate cells of Blood Type B would not fit Type A blood.

North American pokeweed plant, which contains a lectin with the potent ability to stimulate white cell production.

How To Detect Your Harmful Lectins

I often have the experience of a patient insisting that he or she is following the blood type diet to the letter and staying away from all the lectins targeted for his or her blood type – but I know differently. When I challenge the patient's assurance, usually the person will drop all sighs of protest and say in amazement, 'How do you know?'

I know because the effects of lectins on different blood types are not just a theory. They're based on science. I've tested virtually all common foods for blood type reactions, using both clinical and laboratory methods. I can purchase isolated lectins from foods such as peanuts, lentils, meat or wheat from chemical

The Indican Test

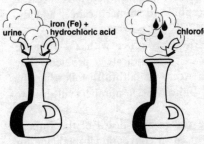

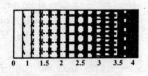

0 1 1.5 2 2.5 3 3.5 4

STEP 1:
Mix urine with hydrochloric acid and iron; the result will be a smoking reaction.

STEP 2:
Let the mixture sit for two minutes, then add three drops of chloroform. There will be more smoke-clear to dark blue in colour.

STEP 3:
Measure colour on the Indican Scale.
0-2   good
2 1/2 problems
3-4   danger

laboratories and the results are visible under the microscope: I can see them agglutinating cells in the affected blood type.

There is a scientific barometer that can be used to measure the presence of lectins in our system. The barometer is a simple urine test called the **Indican Scale**. The Indican Scale measures a factor called bowel putrefaction. When the liver and intestines don't properly metabolize proteins, they produce toxic byproducts called indols. The level of these toxic byproducts is shown on the Indican Scale.

If you avoid foods containing toxic lectin proteins that do not metabolize properly in your system, your Indican Scale will be low.

If, on the other hand, you regularly consume foods that are high in indigestable lectins, your Indican Scale will be high – meaning that you have a high carcinogenity of substances in your body.

My patients with high Indican Scale results often protest that they usually follow the diet, only easing up occasionally. They can't believe that their Indican Scale numbers are so high.

Here's the reason: The Indican Scale shows that a toxic food entering your system is magnified to 90 times the effect on someone for whom it is not toxic. For example, if a Type A eats a processed or cured food, such as bologna (salami), the nitrates are magnified 90 times in the negative impact they have because Type As are particularly susceptible to stomach cancer and the toxic effects of nitrites.

The average person comes into my office with a $2\frac{1}{2}$ on the scale – more than enough toxicity to indicate a problem. The good news is, after only two weeks of faithfully following the blood type diet, that person's Indican Scale number will drop to 1 or even 0.

This may be the first time you've ever heard of the Indican Scale, but it has been widely used in conventional medicine for the last fifty years, and all commercial laboratories perform it. Ironically, only a year ago, several major laboratory groups discontinued its use because not enough people were requesting it. I am certain that as people begin to better understand the blood type-lectin association, the Indican Scale will be revived. Meanwhile, ask your medical doctor or naturopath to perform the test.

A Blood Type Lesson: The Rabbi's Story

Over the years, I have witnessed many transformations as a result of the blood type diet. But few so moved and inspired me as my experience with a wise, elderly Brooklyn rabbi.

In early 1990, I received an urgent phone call from a New York City doctor who respected my work. He asked if I could come to see one of his patients, a renowned Hasidic rabbi who was bedridden. 'Rabbi Jacob is a very special man,' he told me. 'It should be quite an experience for you – and, I hope, for him too.' He went on to tell me that the rabbi, 73, had a long history of diabetes, which was poorly controlled by injectable insulin therapy. Now, a massive stroke had left him partially paralyzed.

When I arrived to see him in his Brooklyn home, I found that Rabbi Jacob was indeed an impressive man who gave off an air of deep spiritual understanding and quiet compassion. Once obviously tall and strongly formed, the rabbi lay withered and exhausted in his bed, his luxuriant white beard almost falling to his chest. In spite of his medical condition, his eyes were clear, kind, and filled with life. His main interest was getting out of bed so he could go about his work. But I could see he was in terrible pain. Even before the stroke, he told me, his legs had been giving him problems. Poor circulation had caused swelling and inflammation in both legs and caused him to experience excruciating jolts of 'pins and needles' when he tried to walk. Now, his left leg was not responding to his bidding.

I wasn't surprised to learn that Rabbi Jacob was Blood Type B. Although this blood type is relatively uncommon in America, it is very common among Hasidic Jews, the majority of whom emigrated from Eastern Europe. I realized that in order to help the rabbi, I must first learn something about the way he lived and the foods he ate. Food was intimately bound to ritual in Jewish tradition.

I sat down with Rabbi Jacob's wife and daughter, both of whom were unfamiliar with naturopathic treatments. But they wanted to help the rabbi, and they were eager to learn. 'He usually eats the same foods every day,' his daughter told me. Those foods consisted of boiled chicken; *chuln*, a type of bean paste; and *kasha*, a buckwheat preparation. Chicken, beans, buckwheat with bow-tie noodles – these are very normal foods. I asked how the *kasha* is made. There was a quick conversation back and forth between mother and daughter in Yiddish, punctuated with lovely smiles at me, and gales of laughter.

'Well,' said the daughter in perfect New York English, 'first you cook up the *kasha* (buckwheat) then you stir it in with the noodles. Then you serve it, say blessings and eat.'

'Do you season the *kasha* at all?' I innocently asked. Another outbreak of Yiddish. Then, the rabbi's daughter began.

'Kasha, Doctor, well . . . you take all the fat you pulled off the chicken while you were koshering it; you put it in a heavy saucepan with just a *bissel* [tiny bit] of chopped onion, and you cook it down. You clarify the fat as it cooks, and you've got beautiful pure chicken fat. We give it to the little ones on a piece of fresh *challah* bread with some salt. It's so delicious you could die!' Yes, yes you could, I darkly thought.

'Anyway,' the rabbi's daughter continued, 'you take some of the *gribbenes*, which is what's left when you cook the fat away. It's all nice and dark and crispy with the caramelized onions, and you put this on the side along with the *kasha* for a little treat. It tastes better than potato chips. The rabbi loves it! The chicken fat you've rendered you mix into the *kasha* and noodles. Oh, it's just delicious. Delicious!'

I learned that these are very common Hasidic dishes, and they comprised the family's typical Sabbath meal. But it was more than just a weekly ritual for the rabbi. A pious man who spent most of his time in prayer, the rabbi thought little of food and simply ate the same meal twice daily, day after day. Although part of a centuries-old tradition, the rabbi's diet was not a good choice for people with Type B blood. The lectins in foods like chicken, buckwheat, beans and corn (not to mention the *gribbenes*!) were causing the cells of his blood to agglutinate, and that was probably a major factor in his stroke. These particular lectins can also block the effects of insulins, which explains why Rabbi Jacob's diabetes became increasingly difficult to control.

I understood that Orthodox Jews obeyed the laws of Kashruth (kosher) ancient dietary principles first laid out in the Old Testament of the Bible. According to these dietary laws, a number of foods are forbidden, and dairy and meat are never eaten at the same meal. In fact, there are separate pots, pans, dishes and cutlery for dairy and meat in kosher homes. And separate sinks to wash all these things, as well.

I therefore approached the matter of dietary changes carefully with the two women, not wanting to disrupt the ritual and religious associations that meant so much. I was also careful not to suggest foods that I knew to be considered 'unclean' in their tradition. Fortunately, there were allowable substitutes. I asked Rabbi Jacob's wife to vary the family diet, restricting the rabbi's typical dishes to once a week for the actual Sabbath meal. For his other meals I asked her to prepare lamb, fish or turkey instead of chicken; rice or millet instead of *kasha*; and to vary the beans used to prepare the *chuln*. Finally, I prescribed several vitamin and herbal combinations to speed his recovery.

Over the next year, the rabbi made wonderful progress. Within eight weeks he was walking and doing moderate exercise, which greatly helped to improve his circulation. He showed remarkable vigour for a man of his age, and shook off the effects of his stroke.

At six months he was switched from injectable to oral insulin therapy – a remarkable achievement considering he had been on injectable insulin for many years. There have been no further episodes of stroke, and Rabbi Jacob's diabetes is finally under control.

Treating the Rabbi gave me a new appreciation for just how ancient and fundamental the wisdom of the blood types is. It also illustrated that foods chosen for religious or cultural reasons may not always be the healthiest for a person of that culture! A five- or six-thousand-year-old tradition may appear time-honoured and ancient, but many of the characteristics of our blood types are thousands of years older.

As you study your blood type diet, take a lesson from the rabbi. The blood type diets are not an attempt to superimpose a rigid formula on your diet, or to rob you of the foods that are important to your culture. Rather, they are a way to fully support your most basic identity – to lead you back to the essential truths that live in every cell of your body and link you to your historical, evolutionary ancestry.

3
The Blood Type Solution: A Road Map

YOUR BLOOD TYPE Plan lets you zero in on the health and nutritional information that corresponds to your exact biological profile. Armed with this new information, you can now make choices about your diet, exercise regimen and general health that are based on the dynamic natural forces within your own body. The next four sections (in Part II) supply highly specific diet, supplement and exercise plans for each of the blood types. These sections are followed, in Part III, by a thorough breakdown of every common health condition and disease, with your particular blood type susceptibilities and remedies. If you follow your Blood Type Plan regime carefully, you can:

- Avoid many common viruses and infections
- Lose weight, as your body rids itself of toxins and fats
- Fight back against life-threatening diseases, such as cancer, cardiovascular disease, diabetes, and liver failure
- Avoid many of the factors that cause rapid cell deterioration, thus slowing down the ageing process

Eat Right 4 Your Type is not a panacea. But it is a way to restore the natural protective functions of your immune system, reset your metabolic clock, and clear your blood of dangerous agglutinating lectins. Depending on the severity of the condition, and the level of compliance with the plan, every person will realize some benefits. That has been my experience, and the experience of my colleagues who use this system, with thousands of patients. It makes perfect scientific sense.

In this chapter I will introduce the elements you will find in your Blood Type Plan. They include:

* The Blood Type Diet
* The Weight Loss Factor
* The Supplement Advisory
* The Stress-Exercise Profile
* The Personality Question

After you read this chapter and review your Blood Type Plan, I suggest you read Part III to get a fuller picture of the specific medical implications your Plan has for you.

The Blood Type Diet

Your blood type diet is the restoration of your natural genetic rhythm. The groundwork for the blood type diets was prepared for us many thousands of years ago. Perhaps if we had continued to follow the inherent, instinctual messages of our biologic natures, our current condition would be very different. However, human diversity and the sweeping forces of technology intervened.

As already discussed, most, if not all, early humans were Type O hunters and gatherers who fed on animals, insects, berries, roots and leaves. The range of dietary choices was extended when humans learned how to rear animals for their own use and how to cultivate crops. But it was not necessarily a smooth and orderly process because not every society adapted well to this change. In many of the early Type O societies, such as the Missouri Valley Indians in North America, the change from a meat-eating diet to an agrarian diet was accompanied by changes in skull formation and the appearance for the first time of dental cavities. Their systems were simply not suited to the newly introduced foods.

Even so, for a long period of time, the traditional agrarian diet provided ample nutrients to avoid malnutrition and support large populations. This changed as advances in agricultural and food-processing techniques began to refine foodstuffs even further, and remove them more and more from their natural state. For example, the refining of rice with new milling techniques in twentieth-century Asia caused a scourge of beriberi, a thiamine-deficiency disease, which resulted in millions of deaths.

A more current example is the change from breast-feeding to bottle-feeding in developing Third World countries. This change to a highly-refined, processed infant formula has been responsible for a great deal of malnutrition, diarrhoea and a lowering of the natural immune factors passed on through the mother's milk.

Today, it is well accepted that nutrition – or the foods we eat – has a direct impact on the state of our health and general well-being. But confusing, and often conflicting, information about nutrition has created a virtual minefield for health-conscious consumers.

How are we to choose which recommendations to follow, and which diet is the right diet? The truth is, we can no more choose the right diet than we can choose our hair colour or gender. It was already chosen for us many thousands of years ago.

I believe that much of the confusion is the result of a cavalier 'one-diet-fits-all' premise. Although we have seen with our own eyes that certain people respond very well to particular diets while others do not, we have never made a commitment – in science or nutrition – to study the specialized characteristics of populations or individuals that might explain the variety of responses to any given diet. We've been so busy looking at the characteristics of food that we have failed to examine the characteristics of people.

Your blood type diet works because you are able to follow a clear, logical, scientifically researched and certified dietary blueprint based on your cellular profile.

Each of the blood type diets includes 16 food groups:

Meat, Offal, Poultry and Game
Seafood
Dairy Products and Eggs
Oils and Fats
Nuts and Seeds
Beans and Pulses

Cereals
Breads, Crispbreads and Muffins
Grains and Pastas
Vegetables, Sprouts, Soya Products and Fresh Herbs
Fruits
Juices and Other Fluids
Spices, Dried Herbs and Flavourings
Condiments
Herbal Teas
Miscellaneous Beverages

Each of these groups divides foods into three categories: HIGHLY BENEFICIAL, NEUTRAL and AVOID. Think of the categories this way:

- HIGHLY BENEFICIAL is a food that acts like a *MEDICINE*
- NEUTRAL is a food that acts like a *FOOD*
- AVOID is a food that acts like a *POISON*

There are a wide variety of foods in each diet, so don't worry about limitations. When possible, show preference for the highly beneficial foods over the neutral foods, but feel free to enjoy the neutral foods that suit you; they won't harm you from the standpoint of lectins, and they contain nutrients that are necessary for a balanced diet.

At the top of each food category, you will see a chart that looks something like this:

BLOOD TYPE O   Weekly portion by ancestry

Food	Portion	African	Caucasian	Asian
All seafood	115–175 g/4–6 oz	1–4x	3–5x	4–6x

The portion suggestions according to ancestry are not meant as firm rules. My purpose here is to present a way to fine-tune your diet even more, according to what we know about the particulars of your ancestry. Although peoples of different races and cultures may share a blood type, they don't always have the same frequency of the gene. For example, a Type A person may be AA, meaning both parents were A's; or AO, meaning one parent was O. Overall, people of Caucasian ancestry tend to have more AA genes; people of African ancestry tend to have more OO genes; and people of Asian ancestry tend to have more BB or AA genes. That is one reason why many people of African descent are lactose intolerant, even if they are Type B (a blood type that benefits from dairy foods).

There are also geographical and cultural variations. For example, people of Asian ancestry are not traditionally exposed to dairy products, so Type Bs of Asian descent may need to incorporate them more slowly into their diets as their systems adjust to them.

These refinements also take into account typical differences in the size and weight of various peoples. Use the refinements if you think they're helpful; ignore them if you find that they're not. In any case, try to formulate your own plan for portion sizes.

At the back of each blood type diet are three sample menus and several recipes to give you an idea of how you might incorporate the diet into your life.

The Weight Loss Factor

Being overweight was anathema to our ancient ancestors, whose bodies were machines which consumed and expended the fuel they needed. Today, obesity has become one of the biggest health problems in many industrialized societies. For this reason, losing weight has become an obsession, and naturally many of my patients are interested in the weight loss aspects of the blood type diet. I always tell them that these diets were not specifically designed for weight loss; they were designed for optimum performance. Having said that, I add that weight loss is one of the natural side effects of the body's restoration. Because the blood type diet is tailored to the cellular composition of your body (as opposed to being a generic, one-size-fits-all recommendation), specific foods will cause weight gain or weight loss for you, even though they may have a different effect on a person of another blood type.

My patients often ask me about current diet plans that are in vogue. The latest are the high protein diets, which have made a recent comeback. By severely limiting carbohydrates, high protein diets force the burning of fats for energy and the production of ketones, which indicate a high rate of metabolic activity. It doesn't surpise me that the patients who tell me they have lost weight on high protein diets are usually Type Os and Type Bs. You don't see many Type As who do well on these diets; their systems are biologically unsuited to metabolize meat as efficiently as Type Os and Type Bs. Nor do Type ABs lose weight on high protein diets, since these diets lack the balance of A-like foods that Type ABs require.

On the other hand, the principles of a macrobiotic diet, which encourage the consumption of natural foods like vegetables, rice, whole grains, fruits and soya, might be best suited to Type As, providing that they eat the recommended grains and pulses.

The bottom line: any time you see a new diet plan that claims to work the same way for everyone, be sceptical. Listen to your blood type. Appreciate your individuality.

* * *

Let me tell you about the weight loss potential of each of the blood type diets. Actually, the greatest problem most of my patients encounter is that they lose too much weight very quickly and I have to make adjustments in their diets to slow down the rate of weight loss. Too much weight loss may seem to be the least of your problems, if you've always struggled with your weight. But remember, your ultimate goal is optimum health and performance, and that means achieving a balance between your weight and your height and shape. Excessive weight loss indicates a malnourished state that will weaken your immune system – exactly what you are trying to avoid. So use these guidelines wisely.

The dynamics of weight loss are related to the changes your body makes when you follow your genetically tailored diet. There are two factors.

First, as your body makes the dramatic shift of eliminating foods that are poorly digested or toxic, the first thing it does is try to flush out the toxins that are already there. Those toxins are mainly deposited in the fat tissue, so the process of eliminating toxins also means eliminating fat.

The second factor is the effects that specific foods have on the bodily systems that control weight. Depending on your blood type, the lectin activity of certain foods may do the following:

- Interfere with the digestive process
- Slow down the rate of food metabolism, so you don't efficiently burn calories for energy
- Compromise the production of insulin
- Upset the hormonal balance, causing water retention (oedema), thyroid disorders and other problems

Each blood type has its own reactions to certain foods; these are outlined in your blood type diet. In the first few weeks you'll need to experiment with the guidelines. I've found that many people approach their diet religiously in the beginning. They eat only the HIGHLY BENEFICIAL foods, and don't even consume NEUTRAL foods. The result is inevitably a rather unhealthy weight loss. They look gaunt and unwell because they're not getting the full range of nutrients needed for a healthy diet. A better approach is to eliminate all the foods on your AVOID list, and reduce or eliminate those NEUTRAL foods that are prone to cause weight gain for your blood type. That will leave you with a balanced diet and a healthier method of weight loss.

The Supplement Advisory

Your Blood Type Plan also includes recommendations about vitamin, mineral and herbal supplements that can enhance the effects of your diet. This is another area where there is great confusion and misinformation. Popping vitamins, minerals, exotic preparations and herbal tinctures is a popular thing to do these days. It's hard not to be seduced by the vast array of remedies overflowing the shelves of your local health food shop. Promising energy, weight loss, pain relief, sexual potency, strength, longevity and mental power – along with cures for headaches, colds, nerves, stomach pain, arthritis, chronic fatigue, heart disease, cancer and every other ailment in the book – these tempting panaceas seem to be the answer we've all been looking for.

But as with food, nutritional supplements don't always work the same way for everyone. Every vitamin, mineral and herbal supplement plays a specific role in your body. The miracle remedy your Type B friend raves about may be inert or even harmful for your Type A system.

It can be dangerous to self-prescribe vitamin and mineral supplements – many of which act like drugs in your body. For example, even though they are all readily available, vitamins A, D, K and B3 (niacin) should only be administered under the care of a doctor.

However, there are many natural substances in plants, called **phytochemicals** (see Appendix C for definition), that are more effective and less damaging than vitamins and minerals. Your Blood Type Plan recommends individualized phytochemical regimens for each blood type.

You may be unfamiliar with the term phytochemicals. Once called weeds or herbs, modern science has discovered that many of these phytochemicals are sources of high concentrations of biologically active compounds. These compounds are widely available in other plants, but in far smaller amounts. Many phytochemicals – which I prefer to think of as food concentrates – are antioxidants, and several of them are many times more powerful than vitamins. Interestingly, these phytochemical anti-oxidants exhibit a remarkable degree of tissue preference, which vitamins do not demonstrate. For example, the milk thistle (*Silybum marianum*) and the spice turmeric (*Curcuma longa*) both have an antioxidant capability hundreds of times stronger than vitamin E, and they deposit with a great degree of preference for liver tissue. These plants are very beneficial for disorders characterized by inflammation of the liver, such as hepatitis and cirrhosis.

Your specialized programme of vitamins, minerals and phyto-chemicals will round out the dietary aspect of your programme.

The Stress-Exercise Profile

It is not only the foods you eat that determine your well-being. It is also the way your body uses those nutrients for good or ill. That's where stress comes in. The concept of stress in very prominent in modern society. We often hear people remark, 'I'm so stressed' or 'My problem is too much stress'. Indeed, it is true that unbridled stress reactions are associated with many illnesses. Few people realize, though, that it is not the stress itself but our reaction to the stress in our environment that depletes our immune systems and leads to illness. This reaction is as old as human history. It is caused by a natural chemical response to the perception of danger. The best way to describe the stress reaction is to get a mental picture of how the body responds to stress.

Imagine you are man before the dawn of civilization. You lie bundled in the dark night, pressed together with your kind, sleeping. Suddenly, a huge wild animal appears in your midst. You feel its hot, rank breath on your flesh. You see it snatch your companion with its powerful claws and tear him apart with its fierce teeth. Do you grab a weapon and try to fight? Or do you turn and run for your life?

The body's response to stress has been developed and refined over thousands of years. It is a reflex, an animal instinct, our survival mechanism for dealing with life or death situations. When danger of any kind is sensed, we mobilize our fight or flight response, and we either confront what is alarming us or flee from it – mentally or physically.

Now, imagine another scenario. You are in bed asleep. All is peaceful and silent. Suddenly, there is a thunderous explosion nearby. Your walls, roof and windows shudder. You are awake now, aren't you? And how do you feel? Probably very frightened and most definitely in some kind of heart-pounding high gear.

Alarmed, your pituitary and adrenal glands flood your bloodstream with their excitant hormones. Your pulse quickens. Your lungs suck in more oxygen to fuel your muscles. Your blood sugar soars to supply a burst of energy. Digestion slows. You break into a sweat. All of these biological responses happen in an instant, triggered by stress. They prepare you – in the same way they prepared our ancient ancestors – for fight or flight.

Then the moment ends. The danger passes. Your body begins to change again. In the secondary, or resistance, stage of stress, your body begins to calm down and compose itself after all of the furore caused by the release of so many chemicals. The resistance stage is usually reached when whatever caused the alarm is identified and dealt with. And then, if whatever caused the initial stress is resolved, all of the reactions disappear, and everything is once again in order within the body's complex response system.

If whatever caused the initial stress continues, however, the body's ability to adapt to the stress becomes exhausted. It shuts down.

Unlike our ancestors, who faced intermittent acute stresses, such as the threat of predators or starvation, our highly pressured, fast-paced world imposes chronic, *prolonged* stress. Even though our stress response may be less acute than that of our ancestors, the fact that it is happening continuously may make the consequences even worse. Experts generally agree that the stresses of contemporary society and the resultant diseases – of the body, the mind and the spirit – are very much a product of our industrialized culture and 'unnatural' style of living. The artificial pressures and stresses of a modern technological society exhaust our built-in survival mechanisms and overwhelm us. We have become socially and culturally conditioned to suppress and thwart our most natural responses. More stress hormones are being released into our blood than we can possibly use.

What is the outcome? Stress-related disorders cause 50 to 80 per cent of all illnesses in modern life. We know how powerfully the mind influences the body and the body influences the mind. The entire range of these interactions is still being explored. Problems known to be exacerbated by stress and the mind-body connection are ulcers, high blood pressure, heart disease, migraine headaches, arthritis and other inflammatory diseases, asthma and other respiratory diseases, insomnia and other sleep disorders, anorexia nervosa and other eating disorders, and a variety of skin problems ranging from hives to herpes, from eczema to psoriasis. Stress is disastrous to the immune system, leaving the body open to a myriad of opportunistic health problems.

However, certain stresses, such as physical or creative activity, produce pleasant emotional states which the body perceives as an enjoyably heightened mental or physical experience.

Although each of us reacts to stress in a unique way, no one is immune to its effects, especially if they are prolonged and unwanted. Many of our internal reactions to stress are ancient tunes being called up and played by our bodies – the environmental stresses that shaped the evolution of the various blood types. The cataclysmic changes in locale, climate and diet imprinted these stress patterns into the genetic memory of each blood type, and even today determine its internal response to stress.

My father has devoted the past thirty-five years to studying the stress patterns and natural energy levels of the different blood types, and devising blood type-specific exercise programmes that draw from the biological profiles of each. In the process, he has observed thousands of people, adults and children alike, and his empirical observations have taken on a valid shape. His findings are remarkably consistent with everything else we know about what makes each blood type function well.

The most revolutionary aspect of my father's work is the discovery that different blood types need different forms of physical activity, or exercise, to cope with their responses to stress.

Your Blood Type Plan includes a description of your own blood type stress patterns, along with the recommended course of exercise that will turn stress into a positive force. This element provides a crucial complement to your diet.

The Personality Question

With all of these fundamental connections at work, it is not surprising that people might speculate about less tangible characteristics that might be attributed to blood type – such as personality, attitudes and behaviour.

I have experienced this personally on many occasions. People often remark about the fact that I have followed in my father's footsteps to become a naturopath. 'You're a chip off the old block,' some will say. Or, 'I guess you've inherited your father's passion for healing'. And sometimes, 'It looks like the D'Adamos have medical genes'.

Even when the observation is made partially in jest, I sense that most people truly believe that I have inherited something besides my physiological characteristics from my father – that it isn't just an accident that I am drawn to the same work that he is drawn to.

The idea that certain inherited traits, mannerisms, emotional qualities and life preferences are buried in our genetic make-up is well accepted, although we aren't sure how to gauge this inheritance scientifically. We don't know (yet!) of any genes for personality. Some might argue that the way we behave has more to do with nurture than nature. But perhaps it is both.

Recently, Beverly, a long-time patient, brought her adult daughter in to see me. Beverly had told me previously that she was young and unmarried when her daughter was born, and she gave her up for adoption. For thirty years, Beverly never knew what had become of her daughter – until the day a familiar-looking young woman appeared on her doorstep, having found her birth mother through a search organization. It turned out that Beverly's daughter was raised on the American West Coast in a very different environment to Beverly's. Yet, I was astounded to watch the two of them together. They were mother and daughter in every way. They possessed exactly the same mannerisms and accents (even though Beverly was a New Yorker and her daughter was a Californian), and they seemed to share a similar sense of humour. Amazingly, Beverly's daughter had chosen the same profession as her mother. Both were human resource managers for their companies. If ever there was evidence of a genetic connection to personality, it was sitting in my office.

Of course, I realize this evidence is anecdotal, not scientific. Most of the research into this aspect of blood types is just that. Still, the connection intrigues us because it makes some sense that there might be a causal relationship between what occurs at the cellular level of our beings and our mental, physical and emotional tendencies as expressed by our blood type.

Evolutionary changes altered the immune systems and digestive tracts of humans, resulting in the development of the blood types. But the mental and emotional response systems were also altered by evolutionary changes, and, with this alteration, very different psychological patterns and behaviours emerged.

Each blood type waged a difficult, and very distinct, battle for its existence a long time ago. The driven loner Type O would have failed miserably in the orderly, co-operative environment of Type A – a big reason for the blood type adaptation in the first place. Would it be such a surprise to find many of these primitive characteristics hidden in some deep remove of our psyches?

The belief that personality is determined by one's blood type is held in high regard in Japan. Termed *ketsu-eki-gata*, Japanese blood type analysis is serious business. Corporate managers use it to hire workers, market researchers use it to predict buying habits and most people use it to choose friends, romantic partners and lifetime mates. Vending machines that offer on-the-spot blood type analysis are widespread in train stations, department stores, restaurants and other public places. There is even a highly respected organization, The ABO Society, dedicated to helping individuals and organizations make the right decisions, consistent with blood type.

The leading proponent of the blood type-personality connection in a man named Toshitaka Nomi, whose father first pioneered the theory. In 1980, Nomi and Alexander Besher wrote a book called *You Are Your Blood Type*, which has sold more than six million copies in Japan. It contains personality profiles for the various blood types – right down to what you should do for a living, who you should marry and the dire consequences that might befall you if you should ignore this advice.

It makes for fun reading and is not unlike astrology, numerology, or other methods of finding your place in the uncertain scheme of things. I think, however, that most of the advice in the book should be taken with a pinch of salt. For instance, I don't believe that a soul mate or a romantic partner should be chosen by blood type. I am Type A and I am deeply in love with my wife, Martha, who is Type O. I would hate to think that we might have been kept apart forever because of some psychic incompatibility in our blood types. (We do just fine, even though mealtimes can be a little chaotic.)

Furthermore, as with all attempts to label people, this one has ominous undertones. Once you say, 'Type A is this' or 'Type B is that' the unavoidable next step is to say, 'Type B is superior' or 'only a Type O can be president'. Caste systems develop. A variation of this happens every day in Japan – for example, when a company advertises that it is looking for Type Bs to fill middle management positions.

So, what is the value of this speculation, and why am I including it here? It's very simple. Although I think the Japanese *ketsu-eki-gata* is extreme, I can't deny that there is probably an essential truth to the theories about a relationship between our cells and our personalities.

Modern scientists and doctors have clearly acknowledged the existence of a biological mind-body connection, and we've already demonstrated earlier in this chapter the relationship between your blood type and your response to stress. The idea that your blood type may relate to your personality is not really so strange. Indeed, if you look at each of the blood types, you can see a distinct personality emerging – the inheritance of our ancestral strengths. Perhaps this is just another way for you to play to those strengths.

The characterizations and suggestions I will make about your 'blood type personality' are based on the pooled impressions made from empirical observations of thousands of people over many years. Perhaps this data will provide a fuller picture of the vital force of blood type. Just don't let it become a source of limitation – rather, let it be a source of *fulfilment*.

By playing to your blood type's strengths, you may be able to achieve greater efficiency and accuracy in your work, and greater emotional happiness and security in your life.

There is as yet not enough hard evidence to justify any sweeping conclusions about the use of blood type to determine personality, but a world of information is waiting to be annexed and explored. A full understanding of the unique cellular blueprint of our bodies still eludes our deepest probing.

Perhaps in the next century we will finally be able to examine some master plan; a map that will show us how to get from here to there within ourselves. But perhaps not. There is so much we don't understand, so much we may never understand. But we can speculate, reflect and consider the many possibilities. That is why we have, as a species, developed such acute intelligence.

* * *

These elements – diet, weight management, dietary supplementation, stress control and personal qualities – form the essential elements of your individual Blood Type Plan. Refer back to the information in this chapter as you familiarize yourself with your blood type.

But before you go any further, I suggest you do one more thing: *Know your blood type!*

PART TWO

YOUR BLOOD TYPE PLAN

4
Blood Type O Plan

TYPE O: THE HUNTER
- Meat-eater
- Hardy digestive tract
- Overactive immune system
- Intolerant to dietary and environmental adaptations
- Responds best to stress with intense physical activity
- Requires an efficient metabolism to stay lean and energetic

Contents

THE TYPE O DIET

Type Os thrive on intense physical exercise and animal protein. The digestive tracts of all Type Os retain the memory of ancient times. The high-protein hunter-gatherer diet and the enormous physical demands placed on the systems of early Type Os probably kept most primitive humans in a mild state of *ketosis* – a condition in which the body's metabolism is altered. Ketosis is the result of a high-protein, high-fat diet with few carbohydrates. The body metabolizes the proteins and fats into *ketones*, which are used in place of sugars in an attempt to keep glucose levels steady. The combination of ketosis, calorie deprivation and constant physical activity made for a lean, mean hunting machine – the key to the survival of the human race.

Dietary recommendations today generally discourage the consumption of too much animal protein because saturated fats have been proven to be a risk factor for heart disease and cancer. Of course, most of the meat consumed today is shot through with fat and tainted by the indiscriminate use of hormones and antibiotics. 'You are what you eat' can take on an ominous meaning when you're talking about the modern meat supply. Fortunately, organic and free-range meats are becoming more widely available. The success of the Type O diet depends on your use of lean, organic meats, poultry and fish.

Type Os don't find dairy products and grains quite as user-friendly as most of the other blood types because the Type O digestive systems have still not adapted to them fully. After all, you don't have to chase down and kill a bowl of wheat or a glass of milk! These foods did not become staples of the human diet until late in the course of our evolution.

The Weight Loss Factor

You will lose weight initially on the Type O diet by restricting your consumption of grains, breads and pulses. The leading factor in weight gain for Type Os is the gluten found in wheatgerm and wholewheat products. It acts on your metabolism to create the exact opposite of the state of ketosis. Instead of keeping you lean and in a high energy state, the gluten lectins inhibit your insulin metabolism, interfering with the efficient use of calories for energy. Eating gluten is like putting the wrong kind of petrol in your car. Instead of fuelling the engine, it clogs the works. I have seen overweight Type Os, who had been unsuccessful with other diets, quickly lose weight solely by eliminating wheat from their diets. To a lesser extent, sweetcorn has the same effect, although it's not nearly as influential as wheat in precipitating Type O weight gain.

There are other factors that contribute to weight gain in Type Os. Certain pulses, especially lentils and kidney beans, contain lectins that deposit in muscle tissues, making them more alkaline and less 'charged' for physical activity. Type Os are leaner when their muscle tissues are in a state of slight metabolic acidity. In this state, calories are used more rapidly. (Before jumping to broad conclusions about other blood types, remember that each blood type has a unique set of factors. Metabolic acidity is not good for everyone.)

A third factor in Type O weight gain is related to thyroid regulation. Type Os have a tendency to have low levels of thyroid hormone. This condition, called hypothyroidism, occurs because Type Os often exhibit insufficient levels of iodine – a chemical element whose sole purpose is thyroid hormone production. The symptoms of hypothyroidism include weight gain, fluid retention, muscle loss and fatigue.

In addition to moderating food portions and choosing leaner meats, for maximum weight control benefits, Type Os need to highlight certain foods for their beneficial or hindering effects. Here's a quick guide:

Foods That Encourage Weight Gain

wheat gluten	interferes with insulin production; slows metabolic rate
sweetcorn	interferes with insulin production; slows metabolic rate
kidney beans navy beans lentils	impair calorie utilization
cabbage Brussels sprouts cauliflower mustard greens	inhibit thyroid hormone

Foods That Encourage Weight Loss

kelp seafood iodized salt	contain iodine; increase thyroid hormone production
liver	B-vitamin source; aids efficient metabolism

red meat
kale
spinach
broccoli $\Big\}$ aid efficient metabolism

Incorporate these guidelines into the total picture of the Type O diet which follows.

Meat, Offal, Poultry and Game

BLOOD TYPE O   **Weekly portion by ancestry**

Food	Portion	African	Caucasian	Asian
Lean red meats, offal and game	115–175 g/4–6 oz (*men*) 60/140 g/2–5 oz (*women & children*)	African 5–7x	Caucasian 4–6x	Asian 3–5x
Poultry and feathered game	115–175 g/4–6 oz (*men*) 60/140 g/2–5 oz (*women & children*)	African 1–2x	Caucasian 2–3x	Asian 3–4x

*Remember: the portion recommendations for all food groups are merely guidelines that can help refine your diet according to ancestral propensities.

Eat lean beef, lamb, turkey, chicken or fish as often as you wish. The more stressful your job or demanding your exercise programme, the higher the grade of protein you should eat. But beware of portion sizes. Our ancestors didn't feast on 450 g/1 lb steaks; meat was too precious and scarce for that. Try to consume no more than 175 g/6 oz at any one meal.

Type Os can efficiently digest and metabolize meats because you tend to have high stomach acid content. This was an essential component in the survival of early Type Os. However, you must be careful to balance your meat proteins with the appropriate vegetables and fruits to avoid over-acidification, which can cause irritations of the stomach lining and ulcers.

One note: Type Os of African descent should emphasize lean red meats and game over fattier, more domestic choices, such as lamb or chicken. The gene for Type O developed in Africa, and your ancestors were the original Type Os. You'll benefit by refining your protein consumption in favour of the varieties of meat that were available to your African ancestors.

HIGHLY BENEFICIAL
Beef, including minced
Buffalo
Heart
Kidney
Lamb
Liver – calf, chicken, pig
Mutton
Oxtail
Sweetbreads
Tripe
Veal
Venison

NEUTRAL
Chicken
Duck
Partridge
Pheasant
Poussin
Quail
Rabbit
Turkey

AVOID
Bacon
Goose
Ham
Pork

Seafood

BLOOD TYPE O		Weekly portion by ancestry		
Food	Portion	African	Caucasian	Asian
All seafood	115–175 g/4–6 oz	1–4x	3–5x	4–6x

Seafood, the second most concentrated animal protein, is best suited for Type Os of Asian and Eurasian descent, as these were a staple of your coastal ancestors' diet.

Richly oiled cold-water fish, such as cod and mackerel, are excellent for Type Os. Fish oils are high in vitamin K, which promotes blood clotting. Certain blood clotting factors evolved as humans adapted to environmental changes, and were not inherent to the blood of early Type Os. For this reason, Type Os often have 'thin' blood which resists clotting. Many seafoods are excellent sources of iodine, which regulates the thyroid function. Type Os typically have unstable thyroid functions, which cause metabolic problems and weight gain.

Make seafood a major component of the Type O diet.

HIGHLY BENEFICIAL

Bluefish
Cod
Hake
Halibut
Mackerel
Red snapper
Perch
Pike

Rainbow trout
Salmon
Sardine
Snapper
Sole
Striped bass
Sturgeon
Swordfish

NEUTRAL

Abalone
Albacore (tuna)
Anchovy
Carp
Clam
Crab

Crayfish
Crocker
Eels
Frogs' legs
Grouper
Haddock

Herring – fresh
Lemon sole
Lobster
Mahi mahi
Monkfish
Mussels
Oysters
Prawns
Red fish

Sailfish
Scallops
Sea bass
Sea trout
Shark
Smelts
Snails
Squid

AVOID
Barracuda
Catfish
Caviar
Conch
Herring – pickled
Octopus
Smoked salmon

Dairy Products and Eggs

BLOOD TYPE O		Weekly portion by ancestry		
Food	Portion	African	Caucasian	Asian
Eggs	1 egg	0	3–4x	5x
Cheeses	60 g/2 oz	0	0–3x	0–3x
Yogurt	115–175 g/4–6 oz	0	0–3x	0–3x
Milk	125–175 ml/4–6 fl oz	0	0–1x	0–2x

Type Os should severely restrict their use of dairy products. Your system is ill-designed for their proper metabolism, and there are no highly beneficial foods in this group's diet.

If you are a Type O of African ancestry, you should eliminate dairy foods and eggs altogether. They tend to be even more difficult for you to digest; indeed, many Africans are lactose intolerant. Soya milk and soya cheese are excellent, high-protein alternatives.

Food allergies are not digestive problems. They are immune

system reactions to certain foods. Your immune system literally creates an antibody that fights the intrusion of the food into your system. Food intolerances, on the other hand, are digestive reactions that occur for many reasons, including cultural conditioning, psychological associations, poor quality food, additives or just some undefinable quirk in your own system. It makes sense that anyone of African descent might be lactose intolerant, since their hunter-gatherer ancestors had no lactose in their diets.

Other Type Os may eat an occasional egg and small amounts of dairy products, but it is generally a poor protein source for your blood type. Be sure, however, to take a daily calcium supplement, especially if you are a woman, since dairy foods are the best natural source of absorbable calcium.

NEUTRAL
Butter
Feta cheese
Goat's cheese
Mozzarella cheese
Soya cheese*
Soya milk*

*good dairy alternatives

AVOID
Blue cheese
Brie
Buttermilk
Camembert
Cheddar cheese
Cottage cheese
Crème fraîche
Edam cheese
Emmenthal cheese
Fromage frais
Goat's milk
Gouda cheese

Gruyère cheese
High- low-fat soft cheese
Ice-cream
Jarlsburg cheese
Milk – skimmed
Munster cheese
Parmesan cheese
Provolone cheese
Neufachâtel cheese
Ricotta cheese
Whey
Yogurt – frozen, Greek-style, with fruit

Oils and Fats

BLOOD TYPE O		Weekly portion by ancestry		
Food	**Portion**	African	Caucasian	Asian
Oils/fats	1 tbsp	1–5x	4–8x	3–7x

Type Os respond well to oils. They can be an important source of nutrition and an aid to elimination. You will increase their value in your system if you limit your use to the mono-unsaturated varieties, such as olive oil and linseed oil. These oils have positive effects on the heart and arteries, and may even help to reduce blood cholesterol.

HIGHLY BENEFICIAL
Linseed (flaxseed) oil
Olive oil

NEUTRAL
Rapeseed (Canola) oil
Cod liver oil
Sesame oil

AVOID
Corn oil
Cottonseed oil
Groundnut oil
Safflower oil

Nuts and Seeds

BLOOD TYPE O   **Weekly portion by ancestry**

Food	Portion	African	Caucasian	Asian
Nuts and seeds	Small handful	2–5x	3–4x	2–3x
Nut butters	15 g/½ oz	3–4x	3–7x	2–4x

Type Os can find a good source of supplemental vegetable protein from some varieties of nuts and seeds. However, these foods should in no way take the place of high-protein meats. They aren't essential in the diet, and should be eaten selectively, as they are high in fat. Anyone trying to lose weight should avoid them.

Since nuts can sometimes cause digestive problems, they must be chewed thoroughly, or used to make nut butters, which are easier to digest. This is especially important for anyone with the colon problems that are more frequently experienced by Type Os.

HIGHLY BENEFICIAL
Pumpkin Seeds
Walnuts

NEUTRAL
Almonds
Almond butter
Chestnuts
Hazelnuts
Hickory nuts
Macadamia nuts
Pecans

Pine nuts
Sesame seeds
Sesame butter
Sunflower margarine
Sunflower seeds
Tahini (Sesame seed paste)

AVOID
Brazil nuts
Cashew nuts
Peanuts
Peanut butter
Pistachio nuts
Poppy seeds

Beans and Pulses

BLOOD TYPE O   **Weekly portion by ancestry**

Food	Portion	African	Caucasian	Asian
All recommended beans and pulses	60–90 g/2–3 oz (dry)	1–2x	1–2x	2–6x

Type Os of Asian ancestry utilize beans well because they are culturally accustomed to them. Even so, beans and pulses are not an important part of any Type O diet. This is because most beans and pulses contain lectins that deposit in the muscle tissues and make them less acidic. Type Os perform best when their muscle tissues are slightly more acidic, as this acidity allows Type Os to burn fat more efficiently. This is not to be confused with the acid/alkaline reaction that occurs in the stomach. In that case, the few highly beneficial beans are exceptions. They actually promote the strengthening of the digestive tract and promote healing of ulcerations – a Type O problem because of their high levels of stomach acid. Even so, eat dried beans in moderation, as an occasional side dish.

HIGHLY BENEFICIAL
Aduki beans
Black-eyed beans
Pinto beans

NEUTRAL
Black beans
Broad beans
Cannellini beans
Chick-peas
Green beans
Lima beans
Peas – green
Sugar-snap beans and peas

AVOID
Kidney beans
Navy beans
Lentils – brown, green, red
Soya beans

Cereals

Food	Portion	**BLOOD TYPE O** Weekly portion by ancestry		
		African	Caucasian	Asian
All recommended cereals	115–175 g/4–6 oz (dry)	2–3x	2–3x	2–4x

Type Os do not tolerate wholewheat products at all, and they should be eliminated completely from the diet. They contain lectins that react both with blood and the digestive tract, and interfere with the proper absorption of beneficial foods. Wheat products are a primary culprit in Type O weight gain. The glutens in wheatgerm interfere with Type O metabolic processes. Inefficient or sluggish metabolism causes food to convert more slowly to energy, and so store itself as fat.

NEUTRAL
Amaranth
Barley
Buckwheat
Cream of rice
Millet – puffed
Oat bran
Oatmeal
Rice bran
Rice – puffed
Spelt

AVOID
Cornflakes
Cornmeal
Cream of wheat
Familia
Farina
Granola
Grape nuts
Wheat bran
Wheatgerm
Shredded wheat

Breads, Crispbreads and Muffins

BLOOD TYPE O   **Daily portion by ancestry**

Food	Portion	African	Caucasian	Asian
Breads, crispbreads	1 slice	0–4x	0–2x	0–4x
Muffins	1 muffin	0–2x	0–1x	0–1x

Obviously, breads and muffins can be a source of trouble for Type Os, since most of them contain some wheat. It may be difficult at first to eliminate morning toast or a daily sandwich; these have become staples of many diets. Even wheat-free breads can be troublesome for Type Os if you eat them often enough; your genetic make-up is not assimilated to the consumption of grains.

The exception is Essene bread, which can be found in some health-food shops. The sprouted wheat version of this ancient bread can be assimilable to Type Os because the gluten lectins (principally found in the seed coats) are destroyed by the sprouting process. Essene bread is a live food with many beneficial enzymes intact.

HIGHLY BENEFICIAL
Sprouted-wheat Essene bread

NEUTRAL
Brown rice bread
Gluten free bread
Millet bread
Rice cakes
100 per cent rye bread
Rye crisps
Soya flour bread
Spelt bread
Ryvita crispbreads
Fin crisps
Wasa bread

AVOID
Bagels
Corn muffins
Cornbread
Durum wheat bread
English muffins
Matzos
Multi-grain bread
Oat bran muffins
Polenta
Pumpernickel bread
Wheat bran muffins
Wholewheat bread

Grains and Pastas

BLOOD TYPE O | **Weekly portion by ancestry**

Food	Portion	African	Caucasian	Asian
Grains	200 g/7 oz (dry)	0–3x	0–3x	0–3x
Pastas	140–175 g/4–6 oz (dry)	0–3x	0–3x	0–3x

There are no grains or pastas that could be classified highly beneficial for Type Os.

Most pasta is made with semolina wheat, so you'll need to select very carefully if you want an occasional pasta dish. Gluten-free pastas made from buckwheat or rice flours are better tolerated by Type Os. But these foods are not essential to your diet and should be limited in favour of more effective animal and fish foods.

NEUTRAL
Buckwheat flour
Barley flour
Kasha
Rye flour
Rice flour
Spelt flour
Quinoa – flour or grain
Rice vermicelli
Rice – basmati, brown, white
Soba (buckwheat) noodles
Tapioca
Wild rice

AVOID
Couscous
Durum wheat flour
Gluten flour
Graham flour
Oat flour

Plain flour
Self-raising flour
Semolina pasta
Spinach pasta
Sprouted-wheat flour
Wholewheat flour

Vegetables, Sprouts, Soya Products and Fresh Herbs

BLOOD TYPE O   **Daily portion – all ancestral types**

Food	Portion	
Raw	140–175 g/5–6 oz (prepared)	3–5x
Cooked or steamed	140–175 g/5–6 oz (prepared)	3–5x

There are a tremendous number of vegetables available to Type Os, and they form a critical component of the diet. Do not, however, simply eat all vegetables indiscriminately. Several classes of vegetables cause big problems for Type Os. For example, the brassica family – cabbage, brussels sprouts, cauliflower and mustard greens – can inhibit the thyroid function, which is already somewhat weak in Type Os.

Leafy green vegetables rich in vitamin K, like kale, collard greens, cos lettuce, broccoli and spinach, are very good for Type Os. This vitamin has one purpose only – to help blood clot. Type Os, as we have discussed, lack several clotting fctors, and need vitamin K to assist in the process.

Alfalfa sprouts contain components that, by irritating the digestive tract, can aggravate Type O hypersensitivity problems. The moulds in cultivated and wild shiitake mushrooms, as well as fermented olives, tend to trigger allergic reactions in Type Os. All of these foods are foreign to the Type O system, which has not been designed to handle them.

The 'nightshade' vegetables, like aubergine and potatoes, cause arthritic conditions in Type Os, because their lectins deposit in the tissue surrounding the joints. Sweetcorn lectins affect the production of insulin, often leading to diabetes and obesity. All

Type Os should avoid sweetcorn, especially if there is a weight problem or a family history of diabetes.

Tomatoes, however, are a special case. Heavily laced with powerful lectins, called *panhemaglutinans* (meaning they agglutinate all blood types), tomatoes are trouble for Type A and Type B digestive tracts. However, Type Os can eat tomatoes. They become neutral in the system.

Type Os can consume all the acceptable fresh herbs liberally.

HIGHLY BENEFICIAL
Beetroot leaves
Broccoli
Collard greens
Dandelion greens
Endive
Escarole
Garlic
Globe artichokes
Horseradish
Kale
Kohlrabi
Leeks
Okra
Onions – red, Spanish, yellow
Parsley
Parsnips
Peppers, red
Pumpkin
Seaweeds
Spinach
Sweet potatoes
Swiss chard
Tapioca
Turnips

NEUTRAL
Asparagus
Bamboo shoots

Beetroots
Broad beans
Carrots
Celery
Chervil
Chicory
Chilli peppers, jalapeño
Coriander
Courgettes
Cucumber
Daikons
Dill
Fennel
Ginger
Green olives
Yicama beans
Lettuce – butterhead, cos, iceberg, Webb
Mangetouts
Mesclun salad mixture
Mung bean sprouts
Mushrooms – abalone, chantarelles, enoki, porcini, Portobello, tree oyster
Peppers – green, yellow
Radicchio
Radish sprouts
Radishes
Rappini
Rocket
Shallots
Spring onions
Squash – all types
Swedes
Tempe
Tofu
Tomatoes
Water chestnuts
Watercress
Yams

AVOID
Alfalfa sprouts
Avocado
Aubergines
Cabbage – Chinese, red, white
Cauliflower
Mushrooms – cultivated, shiitake
Mustard greens
Olives – black, Greek, Spanish
Potatoes – red, white
Sweetcorn.

Fruits

BLOOD TYPE O	Daily portion – all ancestral types	
Food	**Portion**	
All recommended fruits	1 fruit or 90–140 g/3–5 oz	3–4x

Many wonderful fruits are available on the Type O Diet. Fruits are not only an important source of fibre, vitamins and minerals, but they can be an excellent alternative to breads and pasta for Type Os. If you eat a piece of fruit rather than a slice of bread, your system will be better served – and at the same time you'll be supporting any weight-loss goals.

Some of your favourite fruits may be on the avoid list, and some odd choices on the highly beneficial list. The reason that plums, prunes and figs are so beneficial to this blood type is that red, blue and purple fruits tend to cause an alkaline, rather than an acidic, reaction in the digestive tract. The type O digestive tract has high acidity and needs the balance of the alkaline to reduce the possibility of ulcers and irritations of the stomach lining. However, just because a fruit is alkaline doesn't mean it's good for you. Melons are also alkaline, but they contain high mould counts to which Type Os have a proven sensitivity. Most melons should be eaten in moderation, and cantaloupe and honeydew, which have the highest mould counts of all, should be avoided completely.

Oranges, tangerines and strawberries should be avoided because of their high acid content. Grapefruit also has a high acid content, but it can be eaten in moderation because it exhibits alkaline properties after digestion. Most other berries are OK, but stay away from blackberries which contain a lectin that aggravates Type O digestion. Type Os also have an extreme sensitivity to coconut and products containing coconut. Stay away from these and always check food labels to be sure a product doesn't contain coconut oils. These oils are high in saturated fat and provide little nutritional benefit.

HIGHLY BENEFICIAL
Figs – fresh, dried
Plums – green, purple, red
Prunes

NEUTRAL
Apples
Apricots
Bananas
Blackcurrants
Blueberries
Boysenberries
Cherries
Cranberries
Currants
Red dates
Elderberries
Gooseberries
Grapefruit
Grapes – green, purple, red
Guava
Kiwi
Kumquats
Lemons
Limes
Loganberries
Lychees

Mangoes
Melons – canang, casaba, Crenshaw, Christmas, musk, Spanish
Nectarines
Papayas
Peaches
Pears
Persimmons
Pineapples
Pomegranates
Prickly pears
Raisins
Raspberries
Star fruit
Watermelons

AVOID
Blackberries
Coconuts
Melon – cantaloupe, honeydew
Oranges
Plantains
Rhubarb
Strawberries
Tangerines

Juices and Other Fluids

BLOOD TYPE O	Daily portion – all ancestral types	
Food	**Portion**	
All recommended juices	225 ml/8 fl oz	2–3x
Water	225 ml/8 fl oz	4–7x

Vegetable juices are preferable to fruit juices for Type Os because of their alkalinity. If you drink fruit juice, choose a low-sucrose variety. Avoid high-sugar juices like apple juice or apple cider.

Pineapple juice can be particularly helpful in avoiding water retention and bloating, both factors which contribute to weight gain. Black cherry juice is also a beneficial, highly alkaline juice. (You may need to make your own juices if they can't be found in shops.)

HIGHLY BENEFICIAL
Black cherry juice
Pineapple juice
Prune juice

NEUTRAL
Apricot juice
Carrot juice
Celery juice
Cucumber juice
Cranberry juice
Grape juice
Grapefruit juice
Papaya juice
Tomato water (with lemon)
Other vegetable juices (corresponding with highlighted vegetables on page 71)

AVOID
Apple cider
Apple juice
Cabbage juice
Orange juice

Spices, Dried Herbs and Flavourings
Your choice of flavourings can actually improve your digestive and immune systems. For example kelp-based seasonings are very good for Type O because they are rich sources of iodine, key to regulating the thyroid gland. Iodized salt is another good source of iodine, but use it sparingly.

The kelp bladderwrack tends to counter the hyper-acidity of the Type O digestive tract, reducing the potential for ulcers. The abundant fucose in the kelp protects the intestinal lining of the Type O stomach, preventing the adherence of ulcer-causing bacteria. Keep in mind also that kelp is highly effective as a metabolic regulator for Type Os, and is an important aid to weight loss.

Parsley is soothing to the digestive tract, as are certain warming spices, such as cayenne pepper. Note, however, that black and white peppers and vinegar are irritants to the Type O stomach.

Sugar products like corn syrup, honey and processed sugar will not harm Type Os. The same applies to chocolate. But, these should be strictly limited to occasional use as condiments.

Spices, dried herbs and flavourings can all be used liberally if acceptable for Type Os.

HIGHLY BENEFICIAL
Carob
Cayenne pepper
Curry powder
Seaweeds – dulse, kelp (bladderwrack)
Turmeric

NEUTRAL
Agar
Allspice
Almond essence
Anise
Arrowroot
Barley malt
Basil
Bay leaf
Bergamot
Brown rice syrup
Capers
Caraway
Cardamom
Chervil
Chive
Chocolate
Cloves
Coriander

Corn syrup
Cream of tartar
Cumin
Dill
Garlic
Gelatine – plain
Honey
Horseradish
Maple syrup
Marjoram
Mint
Miso
Molasses
Mustard – dry
Paprika
Pepper – peppercorns, red pepper flakes
Peppermint
Pimento
Rapadura
Rice syrup
Rosemary
Saffron
Sage
Salt
Savory
Soy sauce
Spearmint
Sugar – brown, white
Tamari
Tamarind
Tarragon
Thyme

AVOID
Cinnamon
Cornflour
Nutmeg
Pepper – ground black and white

Vanilla – essence, pod
Vinegars – balsamic, cider, distilled white, herb, malt, red and
   white wine

Condiments

There are no highly beneficial condiments for Type Os. If you
must have mustard or salad dressing on your foods, use them in
moderation, and stick to the low-fat, low-sugar varieties.

Although Type Os can have tomatoes occasionally, avoid
ketchup (and brown sauce) which also contains ingredients like
vinegar.

All pickled foods are indigestible for Type Os. They severely
irritate the Type O stomach lining. My recommendation is to
wean yourself from condiments, or replace them with healthier
seasonings like olive oil, lemon juice and garlic.

NEUTRAL

Jam (from acceptable fruits on page 74)
Jelly (from acceptable fruits on page 74)
Mustard
Salad dressing (low fat, from acceptable ingredients)
Worcestershire sauce

AVOID

Ketchup
Mayonnaise
Pickles – Branston, dill, kosher, sweet, sour
Relish

Herbal Teas

The recommendations regarding herbal teas are based on our
general understanding of what makes Type Os sick. Think of
herbal teas as a way to shore up your strength against your
natural weaknesses. For Type Os, the primary emphasis is on
soothing the digestive and immune systems. Herbs like peppermint, parsley, rose-hip and sarsaparilla all have that effect. On the
other hand, herbs like alfalfa, aloe, burdock and cornsilk

stimulate the immune system and cause blood thinning, a problem for Type Os. (You may have to infuse your own herbal teas if they are not located in health food shops.)

HIGHLY BENEFICIAL
Cayenne
Chickweed
Dandelion
Fenugreek
Ginger
Hops
Linden
Lime leaf
Parsley
Peppermint
Rose-hip
Sarsaparilla

NEUTRAL
Catnip
Camomile
Dong quai (Chinese angelica)
Elderflower
Ginseng
Green tea
Hawthorn
Horehound
Liquorice root

Mullein
Raspberry leaf
Sage
Scullcap
Spearmint
Thyme
Valerian
Vervain
Yarrow

AVOID
Alfalfa
Aloe
Burdock root
Coltsfoot
Cornsilk
Echinacea
Gentian
Golden seal

Red clover
Rhubarb
Senna
Shepherd's purse
St John's wort
Strawberry leaf
Yellow dock

Miscellaneous Beverages

There are very few acceptable beverages for Type Os. You're pretty much limited to the innocuous effects of seltzer, club soda and tea. Lager is okay in moderation, but be aware that hops tend to increase stomach acid secretions. Modest quantities of wine are allowed, but it shouldn't be a daily ritual. Green tea (see NEUTRAL Herbal Teas) is allowed as an acceptable substitute for other caffeinated products, but it contains no special curative properties for Type Os. The problem that coffee poses for Type Os is in the increased levels of stomach acid it produces. Type Os have plenty of stomach acid all their own; they really don't need help. If you are a coffee drinker, begin to gradually cut down on the amount consumed each day. The ultimate goal should be to eliminate drinking coffee altogether. The common withdrawal symptoms, such as headache, fatigue and irritability, won't occur if you wean yourself off it gradually.

HIGHLY BENEFICIAL
Soda water
Seltzer water

NEUTRAL
Lager
Wine – red, rosé, white

AVOID
Coffee – decaffeinated, regular
Distilled spirits
Soda – cola, diet, others
Tea – black, decaffeinated, regular

MEAL PLANNING FOR TYPE O

The following sample menus and recipes will give you an idea of a typical diet beneficial to Type Os. They were developed by Dina Khader, M.S., R.D., a nutritionist who has used all the blood type diets successfully with her patients.

These menus are moderate in calories and balanced for metabolic efficiency in all Blood Types. The average person will be able to comfortably maintain weight and even lose weight by following these suggestions. However, alternative food choices are provided if you prefer lighter fare or wish to limit your calorie intake and still eat a balanced, satisfying diet (The WEIGHT CONTROL ALTERNATIVE food is listed directly across from the food it replaces.)

Where herbal teas or fruits are included, check the ones you choose appear on the acceptable lists.

Occasionally you will see an ingredient in a recipe that appears on your AVOID list. If it is a very small ingredient (such as a dash of pepper), you may be able to tolerate it, depending on your condition and whether you are strictly adhering to the diet. However, the meal selections and recipes are generally designed to work very well for each Blood Type.

As you become more familiar with the Type O diet recommendations, you'll easily be able to create your own menu plans and adjust favourite recipes to make them Type O-friendly.

An asterisk (*) indicates the recipe follows.

* * *

STANDARD MENU	WEIGHT CONTROL ALTERNATIVES

Sample meal plan No. 1

Breakfast

2 slices toasted Essene bread *with* butter or organic almond butter 175 ml/6 fl oz vegetable juice banana green tea or herbal tea	1 slice toasted Essene bread *with* natural, low-sugar fruit spread

Lunch

*Organic Roast Beef (175 g/6 oz) *Spinach Salad apple or pineapple slices water or seltzer	*Organic Roast Beef (60–115 g/2–4 oz)

Mid-afternoon snack

*1 slice Quinoa Apple Sauce Cake green tea or herbal tea	sliced carrot and celery sticks sliced fruits 2 rice cakes *with* a drizzle of maple syrup

Dinner

*Lamb and Asparagus Stew steamed broccoli boiled sweet potato mixed fresh fruit – blueberries, kiwi, grapes, peaches seltzer or herbal tea (lager or wine allowed)	steamed artichoke *with* lemon juice *avoid lager and wine*

Sample meal plan No. 2

Breakfast
2 slices Essene bread *with*
  unsalted butter, jam or apple
  butter
2 poached eggs
175 ml/6 fl oz pineapple juice
green tea or herbal tea

1 slice Essene bread *with* apple
  butter
1 poached egg

Lunch
chicken salad – sliced chicken
  breast, mayonnaise, green
  grapes, walnuts
1 slice rye bread or salad greens
2 plums
water or seltzer

grilled chicken breast *with*
  endive and tomato salad

Mid-afternoon snack
pumpkin seeds and walnuts, *or*
rice cakes with almond butter *or*
  figs, dates, prunes
seltzer, water or herbal tea

175 ml/6 fl oz vegetable juice
2 rice cakes *with* natural, low-
  sugar fruit spread

Dinner
*Arabian Fish Dish
*Bean Salad
steamed collard greens tossed
  with lemon juice
green tea or herbal tea
(lager or wine allowed – but not
every day)

*Baked Fish

avoid beer and wine

Sample meal plan No. 3

Breakfast
*Maple Walnut Granola *with*   puffed rice *with* soya milk
  soya milk
1 poached egg
pineapple or prune juice
green tea or herbal tea

Lunch
115–175 g/4–6 oz lean minced   115 g/4 oz minced beef patty
  beef patty   *No bread*
2 slices Essene bread
mixed green salad – cos lettuce,
  parsley, red onion, carrots
  and cucumber
olive oil/lemon juice dressing
water or herbal tea

Mid-afternoon snack
*Carob Chip Cookies (2)   mixed fruit
green tea or herbal tea

Dinner
*Kifta   endive salad
with grilled vegetables   *avoid beer and wine*
brown rice with dab of butter
herbal tea
(lager or wine allowed)

RECIPES

Organic Roast Beef

1 roast beef (about 1.35 kg/3 lb)
salt, pepper and ground allspice, to taste
6 garlic cloves, sliced
extra-virgin olive oil
bay leaves

Preheat the oven to 180°C (350°F) Mark 4. Remove all the
visible fat from the roast and place in a roasting tin. Season and
cut gashes inserting the garlic in the flesh. Brush the meat with
extra-virgin olive oil. Insert the bay leaves. Roast, uncovered, for
90 minutes, or until meat is tender. Remove from the oven and
allow to stand for 15 minutes before carving.

Serves 6

Lamb and Asparagus Stew

225 g/8 oz boneless free-range lamb, cubed
1 medium onion, chopped
salt, pepper and ground allspice, to taste
450 g/1 lb fresh asparagus spears, woody ends discarded, then stalks
  cut into 5 cm/2 inch lengths
juice of 1 lemon

Sauté the meat and onion in a large frying pan until light brown,
using just the fat from the lamb. Add 225 ml/8 fl oz water and
salt and spices. Cover and simmer until tender. Add asparagus
and simmer for a further 15 minutes or until tender. Stir in the
lemon juice and adjust the seasoning if necessary.

Makes 2 servings

Arabian Fish Dish

1 large halibut or cod (1.35–1.8 kg/3–4 lb, rinsed and dried)
salt and pepper, to taste
60 ml/2 fl oz lemon juice

2 tbsp olive oil
2 large onions, chopped and sautéed in olive oil
480–600 ml/16–20 fl oz tahini sauce (see below)
parsley sprigs and lemon wedges, to garnish

For the Tahini Sauce
250 g/9 oz organic tahini
2 garlic cloves, crushed
juice of 3 lemons
2 tbsp finally chopped fresh parsley
2–3 tsp salt

First prepare the tahini sauce. Mix the tahini with the garlic, lemon juice, parsley and salt. Stir in enough water to make a thick sauce. Set aside while the fish bakes.

Sprinkle the fish with salt and lemon juice and let stand for 30 minutes.
    Meanwhile, preheat the oven to 200°C (400°F) Mark 6.
    Drain the fish well and brush with the oil. Place in a roasting tin. Bake for 30 minutes.
    Cover with the sautéed onions and tahini sauce. Sprinkle with salt and pepper. Return to oven and bake for 30–40 minutes until fish flakes easily when tested with a fork.
    Serve the fish on a warmed platter, garnished with parsley and lemon wedges.

Serves 6–8

Baked Fish

1 large piece of cod or other white fish, 900 g–1.35 kg/2–3 lbs rinsed
    and dried
lemon juice and salt, to taste
50 ml/2 fl oz olive oil
1 tsp cayenne
1 tsp ground black pepper
1 tsp ground cumin (optional)

Sprinkle the fish with lemon juice and salt and let stand for 30 minutes.

Meanwhile, preheat the oven to 180°C (350°F) Mark 4.

Drain the fish well and coat with the oil. To prevent fish from drying, wrap it with foil, lightly greased with oil. Season.

Bake for 30–40 minutes, or until fish is tender and flakes easily when tested with a fork.

Serves 4–5

With Stuffing (Optional)

60 g/2 oz pine nuts or flaked almonds
2 tbsp unsalted butter
60 g/2 oz finely chopped fresh parsley
3 garlic cloves, crushed
salt, pepper and ground allspice, to taste

While fish is standing, sauté the nuts in the butter until lightly brown. Add parsley and seasonings and sauté for a further minute. Drain then stuff raw fish with the mixture before coating with oil. *Continue with the main recipe.*

Kifta

900 g/2 lb finely minced lamb
1 large onion, finely chopped
60 g/2 oz fresh parsley, finely chopped
2–2½ tsp salt
1½ tsp each pepper and ground allspice
lemon juice and parsley, to serve

Mix all of the ingredients thoroughly together, using a meat grinder, if you have one.

Using lightly wetted hands, shape the mixture into 7.5 cm/3 inch rolls. Cover and chill until required.

Meanwhile, preheat the grill to high.

Place the kiftas on the grill pan and grill until cooked through, turning them so they brown easily.

Serve hot, sprinkled with lemon juice and garnished with parsley.

Spinach Salad

2 bunches fresh spinach, well rinsed, drained and chopped
1 bunch spring onions, chopped
juice of 1 lemon
¼ tbsp olive oil
salt and pepper, to taste

Place the spinach in a bowl and sprinkle with salt. After a few
minutes, squeeze out all the excess water. Add the spring onions,
lemon juice, oil, salt and pepper.
Serve immediately.

Makes 6 servings

Bean Salad

450 g/1 lb green beans, rinsed, with strings removed and cut into 5
  cm/2 inch lengths
juice of 1 lemon
3 tbsp olive oil
2 garlic cloves, crushed
2–3 tsp salt

Cook the beans until tender in plenty of boiling water. Drain.
When cool, place in a salad bowl. Dress to taste with lemon juice,
olive oil, garlic and salt. Toss well so all the beans are coated.

Serves 4

Carob Chip Cookies

75 ml/2½ fl oz organic canola oil
175 ml/6 fl oz pure honey
1 tsp vanilla essence
1 medium organic egg, lightly beaten
215 g/7½ oz oat or brown rice flour
1 tsp bicarbonate of soda
90 g/3 oz unsweetened carob chips
dash of ground allspice (optional)

Preheat the oven to 190°C (375°F) Mark 5. Lightly grease 2

baking sheets.

Combine the oil, honey and vanilla. Stir in the egg, then stir in the flour, allspice and bicarbonate of soda to form a stiff mixture. Fold in the carob chips. Drop the mixture on to the baking sheets by the teaspoon. Bake for 10–15 minutes until each cookie is lightly browned. Remove from oven and cool on a wire rack.

Makes about 40 cookies

Quinoa Apple Sauce Cake

215 g/7½ oz quinoa flour
140 g/5 oz currants (or other dried fruit from acceptable list)
50 g/2 oz pecans, chopped
½ tsp bicarbonate of soda
½ tsp aluminium-free baking powder
¼ tsp salt
½ tsp ground cloves
115 g/4 oz unsalted butter or 125 ml/4 fl oz organic canola oil
200 g/7 oz Rapadura sugar or maple sugar
500 g/18 oz unsweetened, organic apple sauce
1 large organic egg

Preheat the oven to 180°C (350°F) Mark 4. Lightly grease a 20 × 20 cm (8 × 8 inch) cake tin. Sprinkle 60 g/2 oz of the flour over the currants and nuts and set aside. Combine the bicarbonate of soda, baking powder, salt and cloves with the remaining quinoa flour. Separately mix together butter or oil, sugar and egg. Add the fruit, nuts and apple sauce to the dry ingredients.

Spoon the mixture in to the prepared tin and level the surface. Bake for 40–45 minutes or until a skewer inserted in the centre comes out clean. Cool in the tin on a wire rack, then turn out and slice.

Makes about 16 slices

Maple Walnut Granola

325 g/11 oz rolled oats
1 cup rice bran

140 g/5 oz sesame seeds
75 g/2¾ oz dried cranberries
75 g/2¾ oz dried currants
140 g/5 oz chopped walnuts
ground allspice to taste
50 ml/2 fl oz organic rapeseed oil
225 ml/18 fl oz maple syrup
1 tsp vanilla essence

Preheat the oven to 130°C (250°F) Mark ½. In a large mixing bowl, combine the oats, rice bran, seeds, dried fruit, nuts and spices. Add the oil and stir evenly.

Stir in the maple syrup and vanilla essence until evenly moistened, mixture should be crumbly and sticky.

Spread mixture on a baking tray and cook for 90 minutes, stirring every 15 minutes for even toasting, until the mixture is golden brown and dry. Cool well and store in airtight container.

Serve as required

TYPE O SUPPLEMENT ADVISORY

The role of supplements – be they vitamins, minerals or herbs – is to add the nutrients that are lacking in your diet and to provide extra protection where you need it. The supplement focus for Type Os is:

- Supercharging the metabolism
- Increasing blood–clotting activity
- Preventing inflammations
- Stabilizing the thyroid

The following recommendations emphasize the supplements that help to meet these goals; and also warn against the supplements that can be counterproductive or dangerous for Type Os.

Certain common vitamins and minerals are so abundant in Type O foods that they are normally not needed in supplement form. These include vitamin C and iron, although it won't hurt to take a 500 mg vitamin C supplement every day. Vitamin D supplements are not needed. Some foods are vitamin D fortified, and the best source is the natural light of the sun.

All of these recommendations are based on adherence to the Type O Diet.

BENEFICIAL

Vitamin B

My father discovered that Type Os do well on a high-potency vitamin B complex. There's good reason. Type Os tend to have sluggish metabolisms – a holdover from their ancestors' efforts to conserve energy during periods when food was not readily available. Since modern Type Os experience very different conditions, they don't need this conserving effect, but it remains in the blood type memory. A vitamin B complex can have the effect of supercharging the metabolic processes.

Type Os on the correct diet almost never require special vitamin B12 or folic acid supplementation. I have, however, successfully treated depression, hyperactivity and attention deficit disorder (ADD) in many Type Os by using high doses of folic acid and vitamin B12, in conjunction with the Type O diet and exercise programme. Those vitamins are responsible for the development of DNA.

If you wish to experiment with a high-potency vitamin B complex, make sure it is free of fillers and binders. Improper binding and compressing can make the pill difficult to absorb in your system. Also avoid using a formula that contains yeast or wheatgerm.

Finally, eat plenty of vitamin B-rich foods.

Best B-rich foods for Type Os (*see acceptable lists on pp. 58–81*):
meat
liver, kidney and muscle meats
*eggs
fish
nuts
dark green, leafy vegetables
fruit

*in moderation

Vitamin K
Type Os have lower levels of several blood-clotting factors, which leads to bleeding disorders. Be sure you have plenty of vitamin K in your diet. Since it is generally not recommended as a supplement, pay attention to the foods you eat and choose those that are high in this essential Type O nutrient.

Best K-rich foods for Type Os:
liver
egg yolks
broccoli
green leafy vegetables, such as kale and spinach

Calcium
Type Os should continually supplement their diet with calcium, since the Type O diet does not include dairy products which are the best source of this mineral. With the Type O tendency to

develop inflammatory joint problems and arthritis, the need for consistent calcium supplementation becomes clear.

Calcium supplementation in high doses (600–1100 mg elemental calcium) is probably desirable for all Type Os, but it is especially beneficial for Type O children during their main growth periods (2–5 and 9–16 years), and for post-menopausal women.

Although the non-dairy sources of calcium are not as beneficial, Type Os should employ them as mainstays of their diets.

Best calcium-rich foods for Type Os:
sardines – unboned
canned salmon – unboned
broccoli
collard greens

Iodine

Type Os tend to have unstable thyroid metabolisms, due to a lack of iodine. This causes many side effects, including weight gain, fluid retention and fatigue. Iodine is the key element necessary for the production of thyroid hormone. Although iodine supplements are not recommended, adequate amounts of iodine can be found in the Type O diet.

Best Iodine-rich foods for Type Os:
seafood, especially saltwater fish, (*See list on p. 60*)
kelp
*iodized salt

in moderation

Manganese (*with caution*)

It is difficult for Type Os to get manganese in their diet because manganese is primarily found in whole grains and pulses. For the most part this isn't a problem, and manganese supplementation is rarely recommended. However, a surprising amount of chronic joint pain, especially in the lower back and knees, in Type O patients has been helped with a short period of manganese supplementation. Never do this on your own! Manganese toxicity can result from inappropriate administration, and it should only be used under a GP's supervision.

Herbs/Phytochemicals recommended for Type Os

Liquorice (*Glycyrrhiza glabra*)

The high stomach acid typical of Type Os can lead to gastric irritations and ulcers. A liquorice preparation called DGL (deglycyrrhizinated liquorice) can reduce discomfort and aid healing. DGL should be widely available in health food shops as a pleasant-tasting powder. Unlike most ulcer medicines, DGL actually heals the stomach lining, in addition to protecting it from stomach acids.

Bladderwrack (*Fucus vesiculosis*)

Bladderwrack, from kelp, is an excellent nutrient for Type Os. This seaweed has some interesting components, including iodine and large amounts of the sugar, fucose. As you may recall, fucose is the basic building sugar of the O antigen. The fucose found in bladderwrack helps protect the intestinal lining of Type Os – especially from the ulcer-causing bacteria, *H. pylori*, which attaches itself to the fucose lining the stomach of Type Os. The fucose in bladderwrack acts on *H. pylori* much as dust would on a piece of adhesive tape, clogging the suction cups on the bacteria, preventing it from attaching to the stomach.

I have also found that bladderwrack is very effective as an aid to weight control for Type Os – especially those who suffer thyroid dysfunctions. The fucose in bladderwrack seems to help normalize the sluggish metabolic rate and produce weight loss. (Note, however, that although bladderwrack has a time-honoured reputation as an aid to weight loss for Type Os, it does not work that way for the other blood types.)

Pancreatic enzymes

If you are a Type O who is not used to a high protein diet, I suggest you take a pancreatic enzyme with large meals for a while, or at least until your system begins to adjust to the more concentrated proteins. Pancreatic enzyme supplements can be found in many health food shops, usually in the 4x strength.

AVOID

Vitamin A
Since the Type O's blood is prone to slower clotting, I would not recommend vitamin A supplements without first checking with a GP. These supplements can enhance blood thinning. Instead, take advantage of the rich sources of vitamin A or beta-carotene in the diet.

A-rich foods acceptable for Type Os:
yellow, orange and dark leafy green vegetables (*see list on p. 71*)

Vitamin E
Likewise, I would not recommend vitamin E supplements for Type Os because they also tend to complicate Type O tendencies towards slower blood clotting. Instead, derive vitamin E from foods in the diet.

E-rich foods acceptable for Type Os:
vegetable oils
liver
nuts
leafy green vegetables

TYPE O STRESS-EXERCISE PROFILE
The ability to reverse the negative effects of stress lives in your blood type. As we discussed in Chapter 3, stress is not in itself the problem; it's how you respond to stress. Each blood type has a distinct, genetically programmed instinct for overcoming stress.

All Type Os have the immediate and physical response of their hunter ancestors: stress goes directly to the muscles. The blood type carries a patterned alarm response that permits explosions of intense physical energy.

When encountering stress, the body takes over. As the adrenal glands pump their chemicals into the blood stream, a Type O becomes tremendously charged up. Given a physical release at this time, any bad stress may be converted into a positive experience.

Healthy Type Os are meant to release the built-up hormonal forces through vigorous and intense physical exercise. Their systems are literally suited for it. Exercise is particularly critical to the health of Type Os, because the impact of stress is direct and physical. Not only does a regular intense exercise programme elevate spirits, it enables the Type O to maintain weight control, emotional balance and a strong self-image. Type Os respond well to heavy exercise – in nearly every way.

Type Os who want to lose weight must partake in highly physical exercise. That is because this type of exercise makes the muscle tissue more acidic and produces a higher rate of fat-burning activity. Acidic muscle tissue is in the state of *ketosis* which, as we have discussed, was the key to the success of our Type O ancestors – I'd dare to say that there wasn't an overweight Cro-Magnon on the planet!

Type Os who do not express their physical natures with appropriate activity in response to stress, are eventually over-whelmed during the exhaustion stage of the stress response. This exhaustion stage is characterized by a variety of psychological manifestations caused by a slower rate of metabolism, such as depression, fatigue or insomnia. If there is no change, you will leave yourself vulnerable to a number of inflammatory and autoimmune disorders, such as arthritis and asthma, as well as to consistent weight gain and eventual obesity.

* * *

The following exercises are recommended for Type Os. Pay special attention to the length of the sessions. To achieve a consistent metabolic effect, you have to get your heart rate up.

Mix any of these exercises, but be sure to do one or several of them at least four times a week for the best results.

Exercise	Duration (minutes)	Frequency – times per week
AEROBICS	40–60	3–4
SWIMMING	30–45	3–4
JOGGING	30	3–4
WEIGHT TRAINING	30	3
TREADMILL	30	3
STAIR CLIMBING	20–30	3–4
MARTIAL ARTS	60	2–3
CONTACT SPORTS	60	2–3
CALISTHENICS	30–45	3
CYCLING	30	3
BRISK WALKING	30–40	5
DANCING	40–60	3
ROLLER BLADING OR SKATING	30	3–4

Type O Exercise Guidelines

The three components of a high-intensity exercise programme are the warm-up period, the aerobic exercise period and a cooldown period. A warm-up is very important to prevent injuries because it brings blood to the muscles, readying them for exercise, whether it is walking, running, biking, swimming or playing a sport. A warm-up should include stretching and flexibility moves, to prevent tears in the muscles and tendons.

The exercise can be divided into two basic types: *isometric* exercises, in which stress is created in stationary muscles; and *isotonic* exercises, such as calisthenics, running or swimming, which produce muscle tension through a range of movement. Isometric exercises can be used to tone up specific muscles which can then be further strengthened by active isotonic exercises. Isometrics may be performed by pushing or pulling an immovable object or by contracting or tightening opposing muscles.

To achieve maximum cardiovascular benefits from aerobic exercise, the heartbeat must be elevated to approximately 70 per cent of its maximum rate. Once that elevated heart rate is achieved during exercise, continue exercizing to maintain that rate for 30 minutes. This regimen should be repeated at least three times each week.

To calculate maximum heart rate:

1. Subtract your age from 220

2. Multiply the remainder by 70 per cent (.70). Anyone aged over 60, or in poor physical condition, should multiply the remainder by 60 per cent (.60).

3. Multiply the remainder by 50 per cent (.50).

For example, a healthy 50-year-old woman would subtract 50 from 220, for a maximum heart rate of 170. Multiplying 170 × .70 gives her 119 beats per minute, which is the top level she should strive for. Multiplying 170 × .50 would give her 85 beats per minute, the lowest number in her range.

Active, healthy individuals under 40 and persons under 60 with a low cardiovascular risk, can choose their own exercise programme from among the recommendations listed.

TYPE O: THE PERSONALITY QUESTION

Every person with Type O blood carries a genetic memory of strength, endurance, self-reliance, daring, intuition, and an innate optimism. The original Type Os were the epitome of focus and drive, with a strong sense of self-preservation. They believed in themselves. It's a good thing, too, or we might not be here.

If you are a Type O, you may be able to appreciate this inheritance because the things that make you healthy, inspire you and energize you are very similar to your ancestors'. You're hardy and strong, fuelled by a high-protein diet. You respond best to heavy physical exercise – in fact, you become depressed, despondent and overweight when you are deprived of it.

Perhaps you have also inherited the drive to succeed and the leadership qualities of Type Os – strong, certain and powerful – blushing with good health and optimism.

Former American President Ronald Reagan is a Type O who fits the mould quite well. His administration was characterized by surety, evenness and an unflagging optimism about the future. You never felt that Reagan suffered much in the way of self-doubt. He forged ahead, for good or ill. He was also a risk-taker, in the style of Type Os. People used to call him the 'Teflon president' because he was never felled by the risks he took.

Of course, Reagan didn't exhibit (at least publicly) the sharp, uncompromising, almost brutish style of some leaders. For example, it's not terribly surprising that some famous mafiosos have been Type Os. Al Capone was a Type O. Now there's an example of leadership taken to the extreme. Former Soviet President Mikhail Gorbachev is also Type O, and one of the greatest risk-takers of modern times.

Queen Elizabeth II is a Type O, as is Prince Charles. I find it interesting that the House of Windsor has a history of people with bleeding disorders. Perhaps there's a Type O connection.

5

Blood Type A Plan

TYPE A: THE CULTIVATOR
- The first vegetarian
- Reaps what he sows
- Sensitive digestive tract
- Tolerant immune system
- Adapts well to settled dietary and environmental conditions
- Responds best to stress with calming action
- Requires agrarian diet to stay lean and productive

Contents

THE TYPE A DIET

Type As flourish on vegetarian diets – the inheritance of their more settled and less warlike farming ancestors. If you are an average Type A you might find it too big an adjustment to move away from the typical meat and potato fare to soya proteins, grains and vegetables. Likewise, you may find it difficult to eliminate overly processed and refined foods, since our civilized diets are increasingly composed of convenient toxins in brightly wrapped packages. But it is particularly important for sensitive

Type As to get their foods in as natural a state as possible: fresh, pure and organic.

I can't emphasize enough how critical this dietary adjustment can be to the sensitive immune system of Type A. As you will see in Chapter 9, Type As are biologically predisposed to heart disease, cancer and diabetes. In other words, these are your risk factors. But they need not be your destiny. If you follow this diet, you can supercharge your immune system and potentially short-circuit the development of life-threatening diseases. A positive aspect of your genetic ancestry is your ability to utilize the best that nature has to offer. It will be your challenge to re-learn what your blood already knows.

The Weight Loss Factor

You will be naturally thinner on the Type A diet. If you are accustomed to eating meat, you'll lose weight rather rapidly in the beginning as you eliminate the toxic foods from your diet.

In many ways, Type A is the exact opposite to Type O when it comes to metabolism. While animal foods speed up the Type O metabolic rate and make it more efficient, they have a very different effect on Type As. Perhaps you have already noted that when you eat red meat, you feel sluggish and less energized than when you eat vegetable proteins. Some Type As experience fluid retention as their digestive systems slowly process the unwieldy foods. Type Os burn their meat as fuel; Type As ultimately store meat as fat. The reason for the difference is stomach acid. While Type Os have high stomach acid content which promotes easy digestion of meat, Type As have low stomach acid content – an adaptation of their ancestors who survived on an agrarian diet.

Dairy foods are also poorly digested by Type As, and they provoke insulin reactions – another factor in metabolic slow-downs. In addition, dairy foods are very high in saturated fats, the kind that compromise the heart and lead to obesity and diabetes.

Wheat is a mixed factor in the Type A diet. While Type As may eat wheat, you have to be careful not to eat too much of it or your muscle tissue will become overly acidic. Unlike Type Os who thrive on slightly acidic tissue, Type As can't utilize the energy as quickly, and calorie metabolism is inhibited. This particular food reaction is a good example of the way different foods react in different ways depending on your blood type. Wheat is alkaline in Type Os and acidic in Type As.

In addition to eating a wide variety of healthy, low-fat foods, and balancing vegetables and grains, Type As need to highlight certain foods for their beneficial or hindering effects. Here's a quick guide:

Foods That Encourage Weight Gain

meat	poorly digested; stored as fat
dairy foods	provoke insulin reaction; increases mucous secretions
kidney beans	provoke insulin reaction; slow metabolic rate
lima beans	provoke insulin reaction; slow metabolic rate
wheat (*too much*)	makes muscle tissue acidic; impairs calorie utilization

Foods That Encourage Weight Loss

vegetable oils	aid efficient digestion; prevent fluid retention
soya foods	aid efficient digestion; metabolize quickly; optimize immune function
vegetables	aid efficient metabolism
pineapple	increases intestinal mobility; increases calorie utilization

Incorporate these guidelines into the total picture of the Type A Diet which follows.

Meat, Offal, Poultry and Game

BLOOD TYPE A   **Weekly portion by ancestry**

Food	Portion	African	Caucasian	Asian
Lean red meats, offal and game	115–175 g/4–6 oz (*men*) 60–140 g/2–5 oz (*women & children*)	0–1x	0x	0–1x
Poultry and feathered game	115–175 g/4–6 oz (*men*) 60–140 g/2–5 oz (*women & children*)	0–3x	0–3x	1–4x

*Remember: the portion recommendations for all food groups are merely guidelines that can help you refine your diet according to ancestral propensities.

To receive the greatest benefits, Type As should eliminate all meats from their diet. There are no highly beneficial meats in this group's diet. Let's be realistic, however. The Western diet is still resolutely protein-driven. The trend in fast food restaurants seems to be bigger, and with more fat and calories, than ever before. But, no matter the current trend, I urge you to look at the Type A diet guidelines with an open mind. This way you can begin reducing Type A risk factors for heart disease and cancer in your diet.

Having said that, let me acknowledge that it will probably take time to totally convert to a vegetarian diet. Begin by substituting fish for meat several times a week. When you do eat meat, choose the leanest cuts you can find; poultry is preferable to red meat. Prepare meat by grilling or baking.

Stay completely away from processed meat products like ham, frankfurters and cold cuts. They contain nitrates which promote stomach cancer in people with low levels of stomach acid – a Type A trait.

NEUTRAL
Chicken
Poussin
Turkey

AVOID
Bacon
Lamb
Liver – calf, chicken, pig
Mutton
Partridge
Beef, including minced
Buffalo
Duck
Goose
Ham
Heart
Kidney
Oxtail
Pheasant
Pork
Quail
Rabbit
Sweetbreads
Tripe
Veal
Venison

Seafood

BLOOD TYPE A		Weekly portion by ancestry		
Food	**Portion**	African	Caucasian	Asian
All seafood	115–175 g/4–6 oz	0–3x	1–4x	1–4x

Type As can eat seafood in modest quantity three or four times a week, but should avoid flat fish like sole and plaice. They contain a lectin that can irritate the Type A digestive tract.

If you are a Type A woman with a family history of breast cancer, consider introducing snails into your diet. The edible snail, *Helix pomatia*, contains a powerful lectin that specifically agglutinates and is drawn to mutated Type A cells for two of the most common forms of breast cancer, as you will see in Chapter 10. This is a positive kind of agglutination; this lectin gets rid of 'sick' cells.

Seafood should be baked, grilled or poached to achieve its full nutritional value.

HIGHLY BENEFICIAL
Carp
Cod
Grouper
Mackerel
Monkfish
Red snapper
Rainbow trout
Salmon
Sardine
Sea trout
Snails

NEUTRAL
Abalone
Albacore (tuna)
Crockers
Mahi Mahi
Pike
Porgy
Sailfish
Sea bass
Shark
Smelts
Snapper
Sturgeon
Swordfish

AVOID

Anchovy	Halibut
Barracuda	Herring – fresh, pickled
Bluefish	Lobster
Catfish	Mussels
Caviar	Octopus
Clams	Oysters
Conch	Plaice
Crab	Scallops
Crayfish	Shad
Eels	Shrimp
Frogs' legs	Smoked Salmon
Haddock	Sole
Hake	Squid (calamari)
	Striped Bass

Dairy Products and Eggs

BLOOD TYPE A   **Weekly portion by ancestry**

Food	Portion	African	Caucasian	Asian
Eggs	1 egg	1–3x	1–3x	1–3x
Cheeses	60 g/2 oz	1–3x	2–4x	0
Yogurt	115–175 g/4–6 oz	0	1–3x	0–3x
Milk	125–175 g/4–6 oz	0	0–4x	0

Type As can tolerate small amounts of fermented dairy products, but should avoid anything made with whole milk, and also limit egg consumption to occasional organically produced eggs. This will take some planning, as the Western diet is egg-butter-cream oriented with cakes, pies, biscuits and ice-cream being the big favourites.

Type A choices should be yogurt, kefir and cultured dairy products. Raw goat's milk is a good substitute for whole milk. And, of course, soya milk and soya cheese are excellent substitutes, and are very good for Type As.

Most dairy products are not digestible for Type As – for the simple reason that Type A blood creates antibodies to the primary sugar in whole milk – D-galactosamine. As you'll remember from Chapter 2, D-galactosamine is the essential sugar that, along with fucose, forms the Type B antigen. Since the Type A immune system is designed to reject anything B-like, the antibodies it creates to ward off B antigens will also reject whole milk products.

Type As who are allergy sufferers or experiencing respiratory problems, will be aware that dairy products greatly increase the amount of mucus secreted. Type As normally produce more mucus than the other blood types, probably because they need the extra protection it provides their somewhat too-friendly immune systems. However, too much mucus can be harmful, since various bacteria tend to live off it. An overabundance of mucus inevitably leads to allergic responses, infections and respiratory problems. This is another good reason to limit intake of dairy foods.

HIGHLY BENEFICIAL
Soya cheese*
Soya milk*

Good dairy alternatives

NEUTRAL
Eggs – hen's
Feta cheese
Goat's cheese
Goat's milk
Greek-style yogurt
Kefir
Mozzarella cheese – low-fat
Quark
Ricotta cheese – low-fat
Yogurt – frozen, natural, with fruit

AVOID
Blue Cheese
Brie

Butter
Buttermilk
Camembert
Cheddar cheese
Cottage cheese
Crème fraîche
Edam cheese
Emmenthal cheese
Fromage frais
Gouda cheese
Gruyère cheese
High- low-fat soft cheese
Ice-cream
Jarlsburg cheese
Milk – semi-skimmed, skimmed, whole
Munster cheese
Parmesan cheese
Provolone cheese
Neufachâtel cheese
Sherbet

Oils and Fats

BLOOD TYPE A		**Weekly portion by ancestry**		
Food	**Portion**	African	Caucasian	Asian
Oils/fats	1 tbsp	3–8x	2–6x	2–6x

Type As need very little fat to function well, but a tablespoon of olive oil on salads or steamed vegetables every day will aid in digestion and elimination. As a mono-unsaturated fat, olive oil also has a positive effect on the heart and may actually reduce cholesterol.

The lectins in oils, such as corn and safflower, cause problems in the Type A digestive tract – quite the opposite effect of the beneficial oils.

Of course, there are only two oils that are highly beneficial, and frankly, olive oil is far tastier and better suited for cooking than linseed oil.

HIGHLY BENEFICIAL
Linseed (flaxseed) oil
Olive oil

NEUTRAL
Rapeseed oil
Cod liver oil

AVOID
Corn oil
Cottonseed oil
Groundnut oil
Safflower oil
Sesame oil

Nuts and Seeds

BLOOD TYPE A		Weekly portion by ancestry		
Food	**Portion**	African	Caucasian	Asian
Nuts and seeds	Small handful	4–6x	2–5x	4–6x
Nut butters	15 g/½ oz	3–5x	1–4x	2–4x

Pumpkin, sunflower seeds, almonds and walnuts are all good for Type As. Since Type As eat very little animal protein, nuts and seeds supply an important protein component to the diet. Type As should eat peanuts often because they contain a cancer-fighting lectin. Also eat the peanut skins (the skins, *not* the shells).

If you are Type A and have gall-bladder problems, limit yourself to small amounts of nut butters instead of whole nuts.

HIGHLY BENEFICIAL
Peanuts
Peanut butter
Pumpkin seeds

NEUTRAL
Almonds
Almond butter
Chestnuts
Hazelnuts
Hickory nuts
Macadamia nuts
Pine nuts
Poppy seeds
Sesame seeds
Sunflower margarine
Sunflower seeds
Tahini (sesame seed paste)
Walnuts

AVOID
Brazil nuts
Cashew nuts
Pistachio nuts

Beans and Pulses

BLOOD TYPE A   **Weekly portion by ancestry**

Food	Portion	African	Caucasian	Asian
All recommended beans and pulses	60–90 g/2–3 oz (dry)	4–7x	3–6x	2–5x

Type As thrive on the vegetable proteins found in beans and pulses. Along with the soya bean, and all of its related products, many beans and pulses provide a nutritious source of protein. Be aware, however, that not all beans and pulses are good for Type As. Some, like kidney, and navy beans and chick-peas, contain a lectin that can produce a decrease in insulin production, often a factor in both obesity and diabetes.

HIGHLY BENEFICIAL
Aduki beans

Black beans
Black-eyed beans
Lentils – brown, green, red
Pinto beans
Red soya beans

NEUTRAL
Broad beans
Cannellini beans
Green beans
Sugar-snap beans & peas
Peas – green
White beans

AVOID
Chick-peas
Kidney beans
Lima beans
Navy beans
Red beans

Cereals

BLOOD TYPE A   Weekly portion by ancestry

Food	Portion	African	Caucasian	Asian
All	115–175 g/4–6 oz	6–10x	5–9x	4–8x
recommended	(dry)	3–5x	4–6x	3–5x
cereals	190 g/5 oz (dry)			

Type As generally do well on cereals and grains, and can eat these foods one or more times a day. Select the more concentrated whole grains instead of instant and processed cereals. Introduce millet, soya wheat, cornmeal and whole oats into the diet.

Type As with a pronounced mucus condition caused by asthma or frequent infections should limit wheat consumption, as wheat causes mucus production. Experiment to determine how much wheat you can eat.

Wheat-eating Type As must be sure to balance the intake of the acid-forming wheat with alkaline foods (see fruits). Here we're not talking about stomach acid, but the acid/alkaline balance in muscle tissues. Type As do best when their tissues are slightly alkaline – in direct contrast to Type Os. While the inner kernel of wheat grain is alkaline in Type Os, it becomes acidic in Type As.

HIGHLY BENEFICIAL
Amaranth
Buckwheat

NEUTRAL
Barley
Cornflakes
Cornmeal
Cream of rice
Kamut
Millet, puffed
Oat bran
Oatmeal
Rice – puffed
Spelt

AVOID
Cream of wheat
Familia
Farina
Granola
Grape nuts
Wheat bran
Wheatgerm
Shredded wheat

Breads, Crispbreads and Muffins

BLOOD TYPE A		Daily portion by ancestry		
Food	Portion	African	Caucasian	Asian
Breads, Crispbreads	1 slice	2–4x	3–5x	2–4x
Muffins	1 muffin	1x	1–2x	1x

The Type A guidelines for eating breads, crispbreads and muffins are similar to cereals and grains. They are generally favourable foods, but for anyone who produces excessive mucus or is overweight, these conditions make whole wheat inadvisable. Soya and rice flours are good substitutes. Note that in sprouted-wheat Essene bread (found in health food shops) the gluten lectin is destroyed in the sprouting process. Be aware, however, that some commercial sprouted-wheat breads often contain small amounts of sprouted wheat and are basically wholewheat breads. Read the ingredients label carefully.

HIGHLY BENEFICIAL
Sprouted-wheat Essene bread
Rice cakes
Soya flour bread

NEUTRAL
Brown rice bread
Cornbread
Corn Muffins
Gluten-free bread
Millet bread
Oat bran muffins
Polenta
100 per cent rye bread
Rye Crisps
Spelt bread
Ryvita crispbreads

Wasa bread
Fin Crisps

AVOID
Durum wheat bread
English muffins
Matzos
Multi-grain bread
Pumpernickel bread
Wheat bran muffins
Wholewheat bread

Grains and Pastas

BLOOD TYPE A **Weekly portion by ancestry**

Food	Portion	African	Caucasian	Asian
Grains	200 g/7 oz (dry)	2–3x	2–4x	2–4x
Pastas	140–175 g/4–6 oz (dry)	2–3x	2–4x	2–4x

Type As have a wonderful cornucopia of choices in grains and pastas. These foods are excellent sources of vegetable protein. They can provide many of the nutrients that the Type A is no longer receiving from animal proteins. Stay away from processed products, however, such as frozen meals, prepared noodles with sauces or packaged rice and vegetable combinations; instead, gain the full nutritional benefits from whole-grain products. Bake your own cakes, prepare your own pasta or steam your own rice, using organic ingredients.

HIGHLY BENEFICIAL
Buckwheat flour
Oat flour
Rice flour
Rye flour
Soba (buckwheat) noodles

NEUTRAL
Couscous
Barley flour
Bulgar wheat flour
Durum wheat flour
Gluten flour
Graham flour
Spelt flour
Sprouted-wheat flour
Quinoa – flour or grain
Rice – basmati, brown, white
Tapioca
Wild rice

AVOID
Plain flour
Self-raising flour
Semolina flour
Spinach flour
Wholewheat flour

Vegetables, Sprouts, Soya Products and Fresh Herbs

BLOOD TYPE A Daily portion by ancestry

Food	Portion	African	Caucasian	Asian
Raw	115–175 g/4–6 oz	3–6x	2–5x	2–5x
Cooked/steamed	140–175 g/5–6 oz	1–4x	3–6x	3–6x
Soya Products	175–225 g/6–8 oz	4–6x wk	4–6x wk	5–7x wk

Vegetables are vital to the Type A diet, providing minerals, enzymes and antioxidants. Eat vegetables raw or steamed to preserve their full benefits.

Most vegetables are available to Type As, but there are a few caveats: peppers aggravate the delicate Type A stomach, as do the moulds in fermented olives. Type As are also very sensitive to the lectins in most potatoes, sweet potatoes, yams and cabbage. Avoid tomatoes, as their lectins have a strongly deleterious effect on the

Type A digestive tract. Tomatoes are a rare food called a *panhemaglutinan*. That means its lectins agglutinate in every blood type. However, Type O doesn't produce antibodies to tomatoes, and can eat them, as can Type AB. They're very bad for Type As and Type Bs, though.

Broccoli is highly recommended for its antioxidant benefits. Antioxidants strengthen the immune system and prevent abnormal cell division. Other vegetables that are excellent for Type As are carrots, collard greens, kale, pumpkin and spinach.

Use plenty of garlic. It's a natural antibiotic and immune system booster, and it's good for the blood. Every blood type benefits from the use of garlic, but perhaps Type As benefit most because their immune systems are vulnerable to a number of diseases which garlic ameliorates. Yellow onions are very good immune boosters, too. They contain an antioxidant called *quercetin*.

And, of course, tofu is the staple of the Type A diet. Tofu is a nutritionally complete food that is both filling and inexpensive. Many people in Western societies have an automatic aversion to tofu, however, because it doesn't look very appetizing. Try to purchase tofu that is sold refrigerated, and especially from health food shops where it is likely to be fresher than in supermarkets. Tofu *is* tasteless; it takes on the flavours of vegetables and spices cooked with it. The best way to prepare it is in a stir-fry with vegetables and flavourings such as garlic, ginger and soy sauce.

Fresh herbs that are acceptable can be used in liberal quantities.

HIGHLY BENEFICIAL

Alfalfa sprouts	Globe artichokes
Beetroot leaves	Horseradish
Broccoli	Jerusalem artichokes
Collard greens	Kale
Cos lettuce	Kohlrabi
Dandelion greens	Leeks
Endive	Okra
Escarole	Onions – red, Spanish, yellow
Garlic	Parsley

Parsnips
Pumpkins
Spinach
Swiss chard

Tempe
Tofu
Turnips

NEUTRAL
Asparagus
Avocado
Bamboo shoots
Beetroots
Bok choy
Carrots
Cauliflower
Celery
Chervil
Chicory
Coriander
Courgettes
Cucumber
Daikons
Fennel
Jicama beans
Lettuce – butterheads, iceberg, Webb
Mesclun salad mixture
Mangetouts
Mung bean sprouts
Mushrooms – abalone, chantarelles, enoki, maitake porcini, Portobello, shiitake, tree oyster
Olives – green
Onions – spring
Radicchio
Radish sprouts
Radishes
Rappini
Rocket
Seaweeds
Squash – all types
Swedes

Sweetcorn
Water chestnuts
Watercress

AVOID
Aubergines
Broad beans
Cabbage – Chinese, red, white
Chilli peppers, jalapeño
Mushrooms – cultivated
Olives – black, Greek, spanish
Peppers – green, red, yellow
Potatoes – red, white
Sweet potatoes
Tomatoes
Yams

Fruits

BLOOD TYPE A	**Daily portion – all ancestral types**	
Food	Portion	
All recommended fruits	1 fruit or 90–140 g/3–5 oz	3–4x

Type As should eat fruits three times a day. Most fruits are allowed, although try to emphasize the more alkaline fruits, such as berries and plums, which can help to balance the acid-forming grains that are in muscle tissues. Melons are also alkaline, but their high mould counts make them difficult for Type As to digest. Cantaloupe and honeydew melons should be avoided altogether, since they have the highest mould counts. Other melons (listed as neutral) can be eaten occasionally.

Type As don't do well on tropical fruits like mangoes and papaya. Although these fruits contain a digestive enzyme that is good for the other blood types, it doesn't work in the Type A digestive tract. Pineapple, on the other hand, is an excellent digestive for Type As.

Oranges should also be avoided, even though they may well be favourites. Oranges are a stomach irritant for Type As, and they also interfere with the absorption of important minerals. To avoid confusion let me reiterate once again that the acid/alkaline reaction happens two different ways – in the stomach and in the muscle tissues. When I say that acidic oranges are a stomach irritant for Type As, I'm talking about the stomach irritation they can cause in the sensitive, alkaline Type A stomach. Although stomach acid is generally low in Type As and could use a boost, oranges irritate the delicate stomach lining.

Grapefruit is closely related to oranges and is also an acidic fruit, but it has positive effects on the Type A stomach, exhibiting alkaline tendencies after digestion. Lemons are also excellent for Type As, helping to aid digestion and clear mucus from the system.

Since vitamin C is an important antioxidant, especially for stomach cancer prevention, eat other vitamin C-rich fruits, such as grapefruit or kiwi.

The banana lectin interferes with Type A digestion. I recommend substituting other high-potassium fruits such as apricots, figs and certain melons.

HIGHLY BENEFICIAL
Apricots
Cherries
Figs – dried, fresh
Grapefruit
Lemons
Pineapple
Plums – green, purple, red
Prunes

NEUTRAL
Apples
Blackberries
Blackcurrants
Blueberries
Boysenberries
Cranberries

Dates
Elderberries
Gooseberries
Grapes – black, green, purple, red
Grapes – Concord
Guava
Kiwi
Kumquats
Limes
Loganberries
Melons – canang, casaba, Crenshaw, Christmas, musk, Spanish
Nectarines
Peaches
Pears
Persimmons
Pomegranates
Prickly pears
Raisins
Raspberries
Redcurrants
Star fruit
Strawberries
Watermelons

AVOID
Bananas
Coconuts
Mangoes
Melons – cantaloupe, honeydew
Oranges
Papayas
Plantains
Rhubarb
Tangerines

Juices and Other Fluids

BLOOD TYPE A   Daily portion – all ancestral types

Food	Portion	
All recommended juices	225 ml/8 fl oz	4–5x
Lemon and Water	225 ml/8 fl oz	1x (*in morning*)
Water	225 ml/8 fl oz	1–3x

Type As should start every day with a small glass of warm water into which they have squeezed the juice of half a lemon. This will help reduce the mucus that has accumulated overnight in the more sluggish Type A digestive tract, and stimulate normal elimination.

Alkaline fruit juices, such as black cherry juice concentrate diluted with water, should be consumed in preference to high sugar juices, which are more acid-forming. (You may have to make your own juices.)

HIGHLY BENEFICIAL
Apricot juice
Black cherry juice
Carrot juice
Celery juice
Grapefruit juice
Pineapple juice
Prune juice
Water with lemon juice (*see above*)

NEUTRAL
Apple cider
Apple juice
Cabbage juice
Cucumber juice
Cranberry juice
Grape juice
Other vegetable juices (corresponding with highlighted vegetables on page 117)

AVOID
Orange juice

Papaya juice
Tomato juice

Spices, Dried Herbs and Flavourings

Type As should view these ingredients as more than just flavour enhancers. The right combination of spices can be a powerful immune system booster. For example, soya-based flavourings, such as tamari, miso and soy sauce, are tremendously beneficial for Type As. If you're concerned about sodium intake, all of these products are available in low-sodium versions.

Blackstrap molasses is a very good source of iron, a mineral that is lacking in the Type A diet. Kelp is an excellent source of iodine and many other minerals. Vinegar, however, should be avoided because of its acidic properties.

Sugar and chocolate are allowed on the Type A Diet, but only in very small amounts. Use them as you would a condiment. Minimize your use of white processed sugar. Recent studies have shown that the immune system is sluggish for several hours after ingesting it.

Spices, dried herbs and flavourings that are acceptable can be used liberally.

HIGHLY BENEFICIAL

Barley malt
Blackstrap molasses
Garlic
Ginger
Miso
Soy sauce
Tamari

NEUTRAL

Agar	Capers
Allspice	Caraway seeds
Almond essence	Cardamom
Anise	Carob
Arrowroot	Chervil
Basil	Chives

Bay leaf
Bergamot
Brown rice syrup
Cornflour
Corn Syrup
Cream of tartar
Cumin
Curry powder
Dill
Honey
Horseradish
Maple syrup
Marjoram
Mint
Mustard – dry
Nutmeg
Paprika
Parsley
Peppermint

Chocolate
Cinnamon
Coriander
Pimento
Rice syrup
Rosemary
Saffron
Sage
Salt
Savory
Seaweed – dulse, kelp
Spearmint
Sugar – brown, white
Tamarind
Tarragon
Thyme
Turmeric
Vanilla – essence, pod

AVOID

Gelatine – plain
Pepper – black and white ground, cayenne, peppercorns, red flakes
Vinegars – balsamic, cider, distilled white, herbs, red and white
   wine

Condiments

Condiments are not really recommended for any blood type. Type As in particular should avoid products with pickles and vinegar because of their low levels of stomach acid.

Eliminate ketchup from your diet; Type As can't digest the tomato or the vinegar.

NEUTRAL

Jam (from acceptable fruits)
Jelly (from acceptable fruits)
Mustard – prepared
Salad Dressing (low-fat, from acceptable ingredients)

AVOID
Ketchup
Mayonnaise
Pickles – dill, kosher, sweet, sour
Relish
Worcestershire sauce

Herbal Teas
The Type A reaction to particular herbal teas is exactly the reverse of Type O. While Type Os need to soothe, Type As need to rev up their immune systems.

Most of the health risk factors to a Type A are related to a sluggish immune system, and certain herbs can have a powerful effect. For example, hawthorn is a cardiovascular tonic; aloe, alfalfa, burdock and echinacea are immune system boosters; and green tea produces important antioxidant effects on the digestive tract, providing protection against cancer.

It is also important for Type As to increase stomach acid secretions since they tend to have very low acid levels. Herbs like ginger and slippery elm do this (the latter is available in certain health food shops).

Type As should avoid some of the very herbs that are most helpful to Type Os – like the soothing red clover and cornsilk.

Herbal relaxants, like camomile and valerian root, are perfect fixes for stress. The next time you're feeling stressed, brew a pot of good tea.

HIGHLY BENEFICIAL
Alfalfa
Aloe
Burdock root
Camomile
Echinacea
Fenugreek
Ginseng
Ginger
Green tea
Hawthorn

Milk thistle
Rose-hip
St John's wort
Stone root
Valerian

NEUTRAL

Chickweed

Coltsfoot

Dandelion

Dong Quai

Elderflower

Gentian

Golden seal

Hops

Horehound

Liquorice root

Linden

Mullein

Parsley

Peppermint

Raspberry leaf

Sage

Sarsaparilla

Senna

Shepherd's purse

Scullcap

Spearmint

Strawberry leaf

Thyme

Vervain

Yarrow

AVOID

Catnip
Cayenne
Cornsilk
Red clover
Rhubarb
Yellow dock

Miscellaneous Beverages

Red wine is good for Type As because of its positive cardiovascular effects. A glass of red wine every day is believed to lower the risk of heart disease for both men and women.

Coffee may actually be good for Type As. It increases stomach acid and also has the same enzymes found in soya. Alternate coffee and green tea for the best combination of benefits.

All other beverages should be avoided. They don't suit the

digestive system of Type As, nor do they support the immune system.

Pure fresh water, of course, should be consumed freely.

HIGHLY BENEFICIAL
Coffee – decaffeinated, regular
Green tea
Red wine

NEUTRAL
White wine

AVOID
Lager
Distilled spirits
Tea – black, decaffeinated and regular
Soda – diet, Cola, others
Seltzer water

MEAL PLANNING FOR TYPE A
The following sample menus and recipes provide an idea of a typical diet beneficial to Type As.

See pages 81–82 for the general introduction to meal planning.

As you become more familiar with the Type A diet recommendations, you'll be able to easily create your own menu plans and adjust favourite recipes to make them Type A-friendly.

An asterisk (*) indicates the recipe follows – recipes may occur in more than one of the four diets; if so there will be a page reference.

* * *

STANDARD MENU	WEIGHT CONTROL ALTERNATIVES

Sample meal plan No. 1

Breakfast

water with lemon juice (on rising)	
oatmeal with soya milk and maple syrup or molasses	cornflakes with soya milk and blueberries
grapefruit juice	
coffee or herbal tea	

Lunch

Greek Salad – chopped lettuce, celery, spring onions and cucumber, *with* a sprinkling of feta cheese, lemon and fresh mint	
apple	
1 slice sprouted-wheat bread	
herbal tea	

Mid-afternoon snack

2–3 rice cakes with peanut butter	2–3 rice cakes with honey
2 plums	
green tea or water	

Dinner

*Tofu-Pesto Lasagne	tofu stir-fry with steamed green beans, leeks, mangetouts and alfalfa sprouts
steamed broccoli	
frozen yogurt	
coffee or herbal tea	
(red wine if desired)	

Sample meal plan No. 2

Breakfast
water with lemon juice (on rising)
*Tofu Omelettes
grapefruit juice
coffee or herbal tea

1 poached egg
115 g/4 oz low-fat yogurt with
sliced berries (*see p. 120*)

Lunch
miso soup
mixed green salad
1 slice rye bread
water or herbal tea

Mid-afternoon snack
Carob Chip Cookies (*see recipe
p. 89*)
or yogurt with fruit
herbal tea

*Tofu Dip with raw vegetables
(from acceptable list)

Dinner
*Turkey and Tofu Meatballs
steamed courgettes
Bean Salad (*see recipe p. 89*)
low-fat frozen yogurt
coffee or herbal tea
(red wine if desired)

Sample meal plan No. 3

Breakfast
lemon and water juice (on
   rising)
Maple Walnut Granola (*see*   puffed rice with soya milk
   recipe p. 90) *with*
soya milk
prune, carrot or vegetable juice
coffee or herbal tea

Lunch
*Black Bean Soup   cold salmon with a green salad
mixed green salad   and lemon juice and olive oil

Mid-afternoon snack
*Apricot Fruit Bread   115 g/4 oz natural yogurt with
coffee or herbal tea   a drizzle of honey

Dinner
Arabian Fish Dish (*see recipe   Baked Fish (*see recipe p. 87*)
   p. 86*)
Spinach Salad (*see recipe p. 89*)
mixed fresh fruit with yogurt
herbal tea
(red wine if desired)

RECIPES

Tofu-Pesto Lasagne

450 g/1 lb soft tofu, drained and mashed with 2 tbsp olive oil
140 g/5 oz low-fat mozzarella cheese, shredded, or ricotta cheese
1 organic egg (optional), lightly beaten
2 packages frozen, chopped spinach or fresh, cut up spinach
1 tsp salt
1 tsp dried oregano
750 ml/1½ pints ready-made pesto sauce (you may use less)
9 rice lasagne sheets, boiled and drained

Preheat the oven to 180°C (350°F) Mark 4. Mix the tofu and cheese with the egg, spinach and seasonings. Layer 225 ml/8 fl oz of the pesto sauce in a 22 × 28.5 cm/9 × 13 inch ovenproof serving dish. Layer with the lasagne sheets then cheese mixture and then more sauce. Repeat to finish with lasagne and sauce on top.
Bake for 30–45 minutes until bubbling and golden brown.

Serves 4–6

Turkey and Tofu Meatballs

450 g/1lb ground turkey
450 g/1 lb container firm tofu
60 g/2 oz chestnut flour
180 g/6 oz cups spelt flour
1 large onion, chopped finely
2 tbsp fresh parsley, chopped
2 tsp sea salt
4 tbsp fresh garlic crushed
allowable seasonings to your preference

Mix all ingredients well. Refrigerate for one hour. Roll into small meatballs. You can stir-fry in oil until brown and crisp, or bake in the oven at 180°C (350°F) Mark 4 for approximately 1 hour.

Serves 4

Tofu Omelettes

If you can't find fresh tree oyster mushrooms, soak dried ones in warm water for 25 minutes, then drain well.

450 g/1 lb soft tofu, drained and mashed
5–6 fresh tree oyster mushrooms, sliced
225 g/8 oz red or white radishes, grated
1 tsp mirin or dry sherry
1 tsp tamari soy sauce
1 tbsp chopped fresh parsley
1 tsp brown rice flour
4 organic eggs, lightly beaten
1 tbsp extra-virgin olive oil

Combine all the ingredients, except the oil, in a bowl. Heat the oil in a large frying pan. Pour in half the mixture and cover the pan. Cook over a low heat for about approximately 15 minutes until egg is set and cooked through. Remove from pan and keep warm. Repeat the process and use the remainder of the mixture to make another omelette.

Serves 3–4

Black Bean Soup

450 g/1 lb dried black beans, soaked overnight
2 tbsp vegetable stock
30 g/1 oz garlic, crushed
50 g/2 oz onion, diced
115 g/4 oz celery, diced
50 g/2 oz leeks, chopped and well rinsed
½ tbsp salt
2 tbsp cumin
50 g/2 oz dried parsley
50 g/2 oz spring onions, chopped
1 bunch of fresh tarragon, chopped
1 bunch of fresh basil, chopped

Drain the beans and rinse well. Place them in a large, heavy-based saucepan with 3 litres/5¼ pints water and bring to the boil, skimming the surface as necessary.

Drain the liquid from the beans then add the vegetable stock to the beans and simmer.

Sauté the garlic, onion, celery, leeks and seasonings together. Add this mixture to the beans and continue cooking. Purée 25 g/ 1 oz of this soup for consistency. Garnish with the spring onions, tarragon and basil.

Makes approximately 8 servings

Tofu Dip

225 g/8 oz soft tofu, drained and mashed
225 g/8 oz virtually fat-free yogurt
juice of 1 lemon
2 tbsp snipped fresh chives, or 140 g/5 oz spring onions, chopped
crushed garlic and salt, to season
1 tbsp olive oil
selection of acceptable vegetables from list on p. 117 to serve.

Combine the tofu, yogurt and lemon juice in a blender or food processor at high speed until smooth. If the mixture is too thick to blend well, add a few drops of water. Transfer to a bowl, stir in the chives, garlic and olive oil. Cover and refrigerate.

Serve dip in a glass bowl on a platter of fresh vegetables.

Serves 4–6

Apricot Fruit Bread

300 g/10 oz virtually fat-free yogurt
1 organic egg
140 g/5 oz apricot jam (fruit juice sweetened)
250 g/9 oz brown rice flour
1 tsp ground cinnamon
1 tsp ground allspice
1 tsp grated nutmeg
1¼ tsp bicarbonate of soda

140 g/5 oz dried, unsulphured apricots, finely chopped
140 g/5 oz currants

Preheat the oven to 180° C (350° F) Mark 4. Grease a 22 × 12.5 × 5 cm/9 × 5 × 2 inch loaf tin. Combine the yogurt, egg and jam. Add 115 g/4 oz of the flour and half of the spices plus the bicarbonate of soda. Stir until the mixture is evenly moist.

Stir in the remaining flour and spices. If consistency feels too thick, you can add a few drops of cold water or soya milk to make a thick dropping consistency. Fold in apricots and currants.

Pour the mixture into the prepared tin and level the surface. Bake for 40–45 minutes until a skewer inserted in the centre comes out clean. Remove the bread from the loaf tin and cool on a wire rack.

Cut into slices as required

TYPE A SUPPLEMENT ADVISORY

The role of supplements – be they vitamins, minerals or herbs – is to add the nutrients that are lacking in your diet or to provide extra protection where you need it. The supplement focus for Type As is:

- Supercharging the immune system
- Supplying cancer-fighting antioxidants
- Preventing infections
- Strengthening the heart

The following recommendations emphasize the supplements that help to meet these goals; and also warn against the supplements that can be counterproductive or dangerous for Type As.

BENEFICIAL

Vitamin B
Type As should be alert to vitamin B12 deficiency. Not only is the Type A diet lacking in this nutrient, which is mostly found in animal proteins, but Type As tend to have a difficult time absorbing the B12 they do eat because they lack *intrinsic factor* in their stomachs. (Intrinsic factor is a substance produced by the lining of the stomach which helps to absorb B12 into the blood.) In elderly Type As, vitamin B12 deficiency can cause senile dementia and other neurological impairments.

Most other B vitamins are adequately contained in the Type A diet. If, however, anyone suffers from anaemia, they should take a small folic acid supplement. Type A heart patients should ask their GP about low-dose niacin supplements, as niacin has cholesterol-lowering properties.

Best B-rich foods for Type As (*see acceptable lists on pp 104–127*)
whole grains (niacin)
soy sauce (B12)
miso (B12)
tempe (B12)

fish
eggs

Vitamin C

Type As, who have higher rates of stomach cancer because of low stomach acid, can benefit from taking additional supplements of vitamin C. For example, nitrate, a compound that results from the smoking and curing of meats, could be a particular problem with Type As because its cancer-causing potential is greater in people with lower levels of stomach acid. As an antioxidant, vitamin C is known to block this reaction (although smoked and cured foods should be avoided). However, this does not mean massive amounts of vitamin C are required. I have found that Type As do not do as well on high doses (1000 mg) of vitamin C because it tends to upset their stomachs. Taken over the course of a day, two to four capsules of a 250 mg supplement, preferably derived from rose-hips, should cause no digestive problems.

Best C-rich foods for Type As:
berries
grapefruit
pineapple
cherries
lemon
broccoli

Vitamin E

There is some evidence that vitamin E serves as a protectant against both cancer and heart disease – two Type A susceptibilities. Take a daily supplement, but of no more than 400 IU (international units).

Best E-rich foods for Type As:
vegetable oil
whole grains
peanuts
leafy green vegetables (*see acceptable list on p. 117*)

Calcium

As the Type A diet includes some dairy products, the need for calcium supplementation is not as acute as in Type Os, yet a small amount of additional calcium (300–600 mg elemental calcium) from middle age onwards is advisable.

In my experience, Type As do better on *particular* calcium products. The worst source of calcium for Type As is the simplest and most readily available: calcium carbonate (often found in anti-acids). This form requires the highest amount of stomach acid for absorption. In general, Type As tolerate calcium gluconate, do well on calcium citrate and do best of all on calcium lactate.

Best calcium-rich foods for type As:
yogurt
soya milk
eggs
goat's milk
canned salmon – unboned
sardines – unboned
broccoli
spinach

Iron

The Type A diet is naturally low in iron, which is found in the greatest abundance in red meats. Type A women, especially those with heavy menstrual periods, should be especially careful about keeping sufficient iron stores. However, only take iron supplements under a GP's supervision, so blood tests can monitor your progress.

In general, use as low a dose as possible, and avoid extended periods of supplementation. Try to avoid crude iron preparations such as ferrous sulphate, which can irritate the stomach. Milder forms of supplementation, such as iron citrate or blackstrap molasses, may be used instead. *Floradix*, a liquid iron and herb supplement, can be found at health food shops and is highly assimilable by Type As.

Best Iron-rich foods for Type As:
whole grains
beans – dried or fresh (*see acceptable list on p. 111*)
figs
blackstrap molasses

Zinc (*with caution*)

I have found that a small amount of zinc supplementation (as little as 3 mg per day) often makes a big difference in protecting children against infections, especially those of the ear. Zinc supplementation is a double-edged sword, however. While small, periodic doses enhance immunity, long-term, higher doses depress it and can interfere with the absorption of other minerals. Be careful with zinc! It's completely unregulated and is widely available as a supplement, but shouldn't be used without a GP's advice.

Best Zinc-rich foods for Type As:
eggs
beans and pulses (*see acceptable list on p. 111*)

Selenium (*with caution*)
Selenium, which seems to act as a component of the body's own antioxidant defences, may be of value to cancer-prone Type As. However, cases of selenium toxicity have been reported in people who have taken excessive supplements. Check with a GP before taking selenium supplements.

Chromium (*with caution*)
Because of a susceptibility to diabetes, Type As with a family history of diabetes may be interested in the fact that chromium enhances the effectiveness of the body's glucose-tolerant factor, which increases the efficiency of insulin. However, we know very little about the long-term effects of chromium supplementation, and I would not advise unsupervised use. Type As can best protect themselves from diabetic complications by following the Blood Type Diet.

Herbs/Phytochemicals recommended for Type As

Hawthorn (*Crataegus oxyacantha*)

Hawthorn is a great cardiovascular tonic. Type As should definitely add it to their diet regimen if they or members of their family have a history of heart disease. This phytochemical, with exceptional preventive capacities, is found in the hawthorn tree. It has a number of impressive cardiovascular effects. Hawthorn increases the elasticity of the arteries and strengthens the heart, while also lowering blood pressure and exerting a mild solvent-like effect upon the plaques in the arteries.

Officially approved for pharmaceutical use in Germany, the actions of hawthorn are virtually unknown elsewhere. Extracts and tinctures are readily available through homeopathic physicians, health food shops and pharmacies. I cannot praise this herb too highly. Official German government monographs show the plant to be completely free of any side-effects. If I had my way, extracts of hawthorn would be used to fortify breakfast cereals, just like vitamins.

Immune-enhancing herbs

Because the immune systems of Type As tend to be open to immune-compromising infections, gentle immune-enhancing herbs, such as purple coneflower (*Echinacea purpurea*), can help to ward off colds or flus and may help optimize the immune system's anti-cancer surveillance. Many people take *echinacea* in liquid or tablet form. It is widely available. The Chinese herb huangki (*Astragalus membranaceous*) is also taken as an immune tonic, but is difficult to find. In both herbs the active principles are sugars that act as mitogens that stimulate proliferation of white blood cells which act in defence of the immune systems.

Calming herbs

Type As can use mild herbal relaxants, such as camomile and valerian root, as an anti-stress factor. These herbs are available as teas and should be drunk frequently. Valerian has a bit of a pungent odour, which actually becomes pleasing once you get used to it.

Quercetin

Quercetin is a bioflavonoid found abundantly in vegetables, particularly yellow onions. Quercetin supplements are widely available in health food shops, usually in capsules of 100–500 mg. Quercetin is a very powerful antioxidant, many hundreds of times more powerful than vitamin E. It can make a powerful addition to Type A cancer-prevention strategies.

Milk thistle (*Silybum marianum*)

Like quercetin, milk thistle is an effective antioxidant with the additional special property of reaching very high concentrations in the liver and bile ducts. Type As can suffer from disorders of the liver and gall-bladder. Anyone with a family history of liver, pancreas or gall-bladder problems should consider taking a milk thistle supplement (easily found in most health food shops). Cancer patients who are receiving chemotherapy should consult their GP about taking a milk thistle supplement to help protect their livers from damage.

Bromelain

If you are Type A and suffer from bloating or other signs of poor absorption of protein, take a bromelain supplement, which comes from the enzymes in pineapple. This enzyme has a moderate ability to break down dietary proteins, helping the Type A digestive tract more effectively assimilate proteins.

Pro-biotic supplements

If the Type A diet is new, adjusting to a vegetarian diet may be uncomfortable and produce excessive gas or bloating. A pro-biotic supplement can counter this effect by supplying the 'good' bacteria usually found in the digestive tract. Look for pro-biotic supplements high in *bifidus factor*, as this strain of bacteria is best suited to the Type A system.

AVOID

Vitamin A (beta-carotene)

My father always avoided giving beta-carotene to his Type A patients, saying it irritated their blood vessels. I questioned his observation, as that effect had never been documented. Quite to the contrary, the evidence suggested that beta-carotene may prevent artery disease. Yet, recently studies have suggested that beta-carotene in high doses may act as a pro-oxidant, speeding up damage to the tissues, rather than stopping it. Perhaps my father's observations were correct, at least in the case of Type As. If this is so, Type As may wish to forgo beta-carotene supplements and consume high levels of carotenoids in their diet instead.

One caveat: as we age, our ability to assimilate the fat-soluble vitamins may diminish. Elderly Type As might benefit from small supplemental doses of vitamin A (10,000 IU daily) to help counteract the effects of ageing on the immune system.

Carotene-rich foods acceptable for Type As:
eggs
yellow squash
carrots
spinach
broccoli

TYPE A STRESS-EXERCISE PROFILE

The ability to reverse the negative effects of stress lives in your blood type. As discussed in Chapter 3, stress is not in itself a problem; it's how you respond to stress. Each blood type has a distinct, genetically programmed instinct for overcoming stress.

Type As react to the first stage of stress – the alarm stage – intellectually. Adrenergically charged bulbs flash in their brain, producing anxiety, irritability and hyperactivity. As the stress signals throb in the immune system, they grow weaker. The heightened sensitivity of the nervous system gradually frays the person's delicate protective antibodies. They are too weary to fight the infections and bacteria that are waiting to jump in, like muggers trailing an intoxicated prey.

If, however, a Type A person adopts 'quieting' techniques, such as yoga or meditation, they can achieve great benefits by countering negative stresses with focus and relaxation. Type As do not respond well to continuous confrontation, and need to consider and practise the art of stillness as a calming charm.

If Type As remain in their naturally tense state, stress can produce heart disease and various forms of cancer. Exercises that provide calm and focus are the remedy that pull the Type A from the grip of stress.

Tai chi ch'uan (or *t'ai chi*), the slow motion, ritualistic pattern of Chinese boxing, and *hatha yoga*, the timeless Indian stretching system, are two examples of calming, centring experiences. Moderate isotonic exercises, such as hiking, swimming and bicycling, are favoured for Type As. When I advise calming exercises, it doesn't mean you can't break into a sweat. The key is really mental engagement in the physical activity.

For example, heavily competitive sports and exercises will only exhaust a Type A's nervous energy and make them tense all over again, leaving the immune system open to illness or disease.

* * *

The following exercises are recommended for Type As. Pay special attention to the length of the sessions. To achieve a consistent release of tension and revival of energy it is necessary to perform one or more of these exercises three or four times a week.

Exercise	Duration (minutes)	Frequency – times per week
T'AI CHI	30–45	3–5
HATHA YOGA	30	3–5
MARTIAL ARTS	60	2–3
GOLF	60	2–3
CYCLING	60	2–3
BRISK WALKING	20–40	2–3
HIKING	40–60	2–3
SWIMMING	30	3–4
DANCING	30–45	2–3
AEROBICS (low impact)	30–45	2–3
STRETCHING	15	3–5

Type A Exercise Guidelines

T'ai Chi

Tai chi ch'uan (or *t'ai chi*), is an exercise that enhances the flexibility of body movement. The slow, graceful, elegant gestures of the routines mask the full-speed hand and foot blows, blocks and parries they represent. In China, *t'ai chi* is practised daily by groups who gather in parks and public squares to perform the movements in unison. *T'ai chi* can be a very effective relaxation technique, although it takes concentration and patience to master.

Yoga

Yoga is also good for the Type A stress pattern. It combines inner rectitude with breath control and postures designed to allow complete concentration without distraction by worldly concerns. *Hatha yoga* is the most common form of yoga practised in the West.

After learning basic yoga postures, one can create a routine best suited for an individual lifestyle. Many Type As who have adopted yoga relaxation tell me they will not leave the house until they have done their yoga.

However, some patients have told me that they are concerned

that adopting yoga practices may conflict with their religious beliefs. They fear it implies they have adopted Eastern mysticism. I respond, 'If you eat Italian food, does that make you Italian?' Meditation and yoga are what you make them. Visualize and meditate on those subjects which are relevant to you. The postures are neutral – they are just timeless and proven movements.

Simple yoga relaxation techniques

Yoga begins and ends with relaxation. We contract our muscles constantly, but rarely do we think of doing the opposite – letting go and relaxing. We can feel better and be healthier if we regularly release the tensions left behind within the muscles by the stresses and strains of life.

The best position for relaxation is lying on your back. Arrange your arms and legs so you are comfortable in your hips, shoulders and back. The goal of deep relaxation is to let your body and mind settle down to soothing calmness, in the same way that an agitated pool of water eventually calms down to stillness.

Begin with abdominal breathing. As a baby breathes, its abdomen moves, not its chest. However, many of us grow to unconsciously adopt the unnatural and inefficient habit of restrained chest breathing. One of the aims of yoga is to make you aware of the true centre of breathing.

Observe the pattern of your breathing. Is your breathing fast, shallow, irregular, or do you tend to hold your breath? Allow your breathing to revert to a more natural pattern – full, deep, regular and with no constriction. Try to isolate just your lower breathing muscles; see if you can breathe without moving your chest. Breathing exercises are always done smoothly and without any strain. Place one hand on your navel and feel the movement of your breathing. Relax your shoulders.

Start the exercise by breathing out completely. When you inhale, pretend that a heavy weight, such as a large book, is resting on your navel, and that by your inhalation, you are trying to raise this imaginary weight up towards the ceiling.

Then when you exhale, simply let this imaginary weight press down against your abdomen, helping you to exhale. Exhale more air than you normally would, as if to 'squeeze' more air out of your lungs. This will act as a yoga stretch for the diaphragm and help to release tension in this muscle.

Bring your abdominal muscles into play here to assist. When you inhale, direct your breath down so deeply that you are lifting the imaginary heavy weight back up towards the ceiling. Try to completely co-ordinate and isolate the abdominal breath with no chest or rib movement.

Even if you perform exercises that are more aerobic during the week, try to integrate with the relaxing, soothing routines that will help you best manage your Type A stress patterns.

TYPE A: THE PERSONALITY QUESTION

Blood Type A was originally adapted to deal with dense population concentrations and the stresses of a more sedentary but intense urban lifestyle. Certain psychological traits would develop in people who must tolerate the demands of a crowded environment.

Probably the most important quality a person must have in that setting is a co-operative nature. The original Type As had to be decent, orderly, law-abiding and exhibit self-control. Communities can't exist without respect for others and their property. Loners do poorly in group settings. If the characteristics of Type Os had not evolved to suit an agrarian society, the result would have been chaos – and ultimately doom. Again, it's thanks to our Type A ancestors that humans survived.

The early Type As had to be clever, sensitive, passionate and very smart to meet the challenges of a more complex life. But all of these qualities had to exist within a framework. That may be the reason why Type As, even today, tend to have more tightly wired systems. They bottle up their anxiety – because that's what you do when you're trying to get along with others – but when they explode, watch out! The antidote to this tremendous inner stress is, as I have discussed, the more soothing and contemplative relaxation exercises of yoga and *t'ai chi*.

It would seem that Type As are poorly suited for the intense, highly-pressured leadership positions at which Type Os excel.

That's not to say they can't be leaders. But they instinctively reject the dog-eat-dog manner of contemporary leadership. When Type As get into these positions, they tend to unravel. Former American presidents Lyndon Johnson, Richard Nixon and Jimmy Carter were all Type A. While each man brought an unquestioned brilliance and passion to the job, all of them possessed fatal flaws. When the stress got too great, they became anxious and paranoid, taking everything personally. In the end, it was these Type A responses that forced each of them out of office.

Perhaps the most well-known Type A was Adolf Hitler. While most people might associate him with the sheer drive and brutal surety of the Type O leader, Hitler's overriding trait was really an extraordinary hypersensitivity that led him ultimately to madness. Hitler was an anomalous being. His obsession with a genetically ordered society was that of a mutated Type A personality with a nightmarish vision.

6
Blood Type B Plan

```
TYPE B: THE NOMAD
• Balanced
• Strong immune system
• Tolerant digestive system
• Most flexible dietary choices
• Diary eater
• Responds best to stress with creativity
• Requires a balance between physical and mental activity
    to stay lean and sharp
```

Contents

THE TYPE B DIET

Type O and Type A seem to be polar opposites in many respects. But Type B can best be described as idiosyncratic – with utterly unique and sometimes chameleon-like characteristics. In many respects, Type B resembles Type O so much that the two seem related. Then, suddenly, Type B will take on a totally unfamiliar shape – one that is peculiarly its own. You might say Type B represents a sophisticated refinement in the evolutionary journey, an effort to join together divergent peoples and cultures.

On the whole, the sturdy and alert Type Bs are usually able to resist many of the most severe diseases common to modern life, such as heart disease and cancer. Even when they do contract these diseases, they are more likely to survive them. Yet, because Type B is somewhat off beat, its system seems more prone to less common immune system disorders, such as Chronic Fatigue Syndrome (ME), Multiple Sclerosis, and lupus (see Chapter 9).

In my experience, a Type B who carefully follows the recommended diet can often bypass severe disease and live a long and healthy life.

The Type B diet is balanced and wholesome, including a wide variety of foods. In the words of my father, it represents 'the best of the animal and vegetable kingdoms'. Think of B as standing for balance – the balancing forces of A and O.

The Weight Loss Factor

For Type Bs, the biggest factors in weight gain are corn, buckwheat, lentils, peanuts and sesame seeds. Each of these foods has a different lectin, but all of them affect insulin production, resulting in fatigue, fluid retention and hypoglycaemia – a severe drop in blood sugar after eating a meal.

Type Bs are similar to Type Os in their reaction to the gluten found in wheatgerm and wholewheat products. The gluten lectin adds to the problems caused by the other metabolism–slowing foods. When food is not efficiently digested and burned as fuel for the body, it gets stored as fat. In itself, the wheat gluten doesn't attack Type Bs as severely as it does Type Os. However, when you add wheat to the mix of corn, lentils, buckwheat and peanuts, the end result is just as damaging. Type Bs who want to lose weight should definitely avoid wheat.

When these foods are avoided, along with others that contain toxic lectins, it has been my experience that Type Bs are very successful in controlling their weight. They don't have any natural physiological barriers to weight loss, such as the thyroid problems that can hamper Type Os. Nor do they suffer from digestive disorders. All that's necessary to lose weight is to stay on the diet.

Some people are surprised that Type Bs aren't more likely to have problems with weight control, since dairy foods are encouraged on the diet. Of course, if you overeat high-calorie foods, you're going to gain weight! But a moderate consumption of dairy foods actually helps Type Bs achieve a metabolic balance. The real culprits are the particular foods that inhibit the efficient use of energy and promote the storage of calories as fat.

These are the highlights for Type B weight loss:

Foods That Encourage Weight Gain

sweetcorn	inhibits insulin production; hampers metabolic rate
lentils	cause hypoglycaemia inhibit proper nutrient uptake hamper metabolic efficiency
peanuts	hamper metabolic efficiency cause hypoglycaemia inhibit liver function
sesame seeds	hamper metabolic efficiency cause hypoglycaemia
buckwheat	inhibits digestion hampers metabolic efficiency causes hypoglycaemia
wheat	slows the digestive and metabolic processes; causes food to be stored as fat, not burned as energy

Foods That Encourage Weight Loss

green vegetables meat liver eggs	aid efficient metabolism
liquorice tea [†]	counters hypoglycaemia

([†] Note: *Never take liquorice supplements without a GP's supervision; liquorice tea is OK.*)

Incorporate these guidelines into the total picture of the Type B Diet that follows.

Meat, Offal, Poultry and Game

BLOOD TYPE B   **Weekly portion by ancestry**

Food	Portion	African	Caucasian	Asian
Lean red meats, offal and game	115–175 g/4–6 oz (*men*) 60–140 g/2–5 oz (*women and children*)	3–4x	2–3x	2–3x
Poultry and feathered game	115–175 g/4–6 oz (*men*) 60–140 g/2–5 oz (*women and children*)	0–2x	0–3x	0–2x

Remember: the portion recommendations for all food groups are merely guidelines that can help you refine your diet according to ancestral propensities.

There appears to be a direct connection between stress, autoimmune disorders and red meat in the Type B system. That's because Type B ancestors adapted better to other kinds of meats. Any Type B who is fatigued or suffering from immune deficiencies should eat lamb, mutton or rabbit several times a week, in preference to beef or turkey.

In my experience, one of the most difficult adjustments Type Bs must make is to give up chicken. Chicken contains a Blood Type B agglutinating lectin in its muscle tissue. Anyone accustomed to eating more poultry than red meat can eat other poultry or game, such as turkey or pheasant. Although they are similar to chicken in many respects, neither contains the dangerous lectin.

The news about chicken is troubling to many people because chicken has become a fundamental part of many ethnic diets. In addition, people have been told to eat chicken instead of beef because it is 'healthier'. But here is another case where one dietary guideline does not fit all. Chicken may be leaner (although not always) than other meat, but that isn't the issue. The issue is the power of an agglutinating lectin to attack the bloodstream and potentially lead to strokes and immune disorders. So, even though chicken may be a beloved food, I urge you to wean yourself away from it.

HIGHLY BENEFICIAL
Lamb
Mutton
Rabbit
Venison

NEUTRAL
Beef, including minced
Liver – calf, chicken, pig
Pheasant
Turkey
Veal

AVOID
Bacon
Chicken
Duck
Goose
Ham
Heart
Partridge
Pork
Poussin
Quail

Seafood

BLOOD TYPE B   **Weekly portion by ancestry**

Food All seafood	Portion 115–175 g/4–6 oz	African 4–6x	Caucasian 3–5x	Asian 3–5x

Type Bs thrive on seafood, especially the deep-sea fish like cod and salmon, which are rich in nutritious oils. White fish, such as cod, halibut and sole, are excellent sources of high-quality protein for Type Bs. Avoid all shellfish – crab, lobster, prawns, mussels, etc. They contain lectins that are disruptive to the Type B system. It is interesting to note that many of the original Type Bs were Jewish tribes that forbade the consumption of shellfish. Perhaps this dietary law was an acknowledgement that shellfish are poorly digested by Type Bs.

HIGHLY BENEFICIAL

Cod	Pike
Grouper	Porgy
Haddock	Red Fish
Hake	Sardines
Halibut	Sea trout
Mackerel	Shad
Mahi mahi	Sturgeon
Monkfish	

NEUTRAL

Abalone	Rainbow trout
Albacore (tuna)	Sailfish
Bluefish	Salmon
Carp	Scallop
Catfish	Shark
Caviar	Smelts
Crockers	Snapper
Herring – fresh, pickled	Sole
Mussels	Squid
Red snapper	Swordfish

AVOID

Anchovy	Lobster
Barracuda	Octopus
Clams	Oysters
Conch	Prawns
Crab	Sea Bass
Crayfish	Smoked salmon
Eels	Snails
Frogs' legs	Striped bass

Dairy Products and Eggs

BLOOD TYPE B		Weekly portion by ancestry		
Food	Portion	African	Caucasian	Asian
Eggs	1 egg	3–4x	3–4x	5–6x
Cheeses	60 g/2 oz	3–4x	3–5x	2–3x
Yogurt	115–175 g/4–6 oz	0–4x	2–4x	1–3x
Milk	125–175 g/4–6 fl oz	0–3x	4–5x	2–3x

Type B is the only blood type that can fully enjoy a variety of dairy foods. That's because the primary sugar in the Type B antigen is D-galactosamine, the same sugar present in milk. Dairy foods were first introduced to the human diet during the height of the Type B development, along with the domestication of animals. (By the way, eggs do not contain the lectin that is found in the muscle tissues of chicken.)

However, there are ancestral idiosyncracies that blur the picture. Any Type A of Asian descent may initially have a problem adapting to dairy foods – not because your system is resistant to them, but because your culture has typically been resistant. Dairy products were first introduced into Asian societies with the invasion of the Mongolian hordes. To the Asian mind, dairy products were the food of the barbarian, and thus not fit to eat. The stigma remains to this day, although there are large numbers of Type Bs in Asia whose soya-based diet is damaging to their systems.

Type Bs of African descent might also have trouble adapting

to dairy foods. Type Bs are barely represented in Africa, and many Africans are lactose intolerant.

These intolerances should not be confused with allergies. Allergies are immune responses that cause blood to produce an antibody to a food. Intolerances are digestive problems with certain foods. Intolerances are caused by migration, cultural assimilation and other factors – for example, when Type Bs moved into Africa where dairy foods were not prominent.

What can you do? If you are lactose intolerant, begin using a lactose enzyme preparation, which will make digestion of dairy foods possible. Then, after following the Type B diet for several weeks, slowly introduce dairy foods – beginning with cultured or soured dairy products, such as buttermilk, yogurt and kefir, which may be better tolerated than fresh milk products, such as ice-cream, whole milk and high-fat soft cheese. I've found that lactose intolerant Type Bs are often able to incorporate dairy foods after they have corrected the overall problems in their diets.

Soya foods are often recommended as dairy substitutes, although they're mostly benign for Type Bs. They don't have the many health benefits for Type Bs that they have for Type As. Part of my concern about recommending soya for Type Bs is the danger that people will substitute them too often as main courses, instead of eating the meat, fish and dairy products that Type Bs really need for optimum health.

HIGHLY BENEFICIAL
Cottage cheese
Feta cheese
Goat's cheese
Goat's milk
Kefir
Milk – skimmed, semi-skimmed
Mozzarella cheese
Ricotta cheese
Yogurt – frozen, Greek-style, with fruit

NEUTRAL
Brie
Butter
Buttermilk
Camembert
Cheddar cheese
Crème fraîche
Edam cheese
Emmenthal cheese
Fromage frais
Gouda cheese
Gruyère cheese
High-/low-fat soft cheese
Jarlsburg cheese
Milk – whole
Munster cheese
Neufachâtel cheese
Quark
Parmesan cheese
Provolone cheese
Sherbet
Soya milk
Whey

AVOID
Blue cheese
Ice-cream

Oils and Fats

BLOOD TYPE B		Weekly portion by ancestry		
Food	Portion	African	Caucasian	Asian
Oils/fats	1 tbsp	3–5x	4–6x	5–7x

Introduce olive oil into your diet to encourage proper digestion and healthy elimination. Use at least one tablespoon every other day. Ghee, an Indian preparation similar to clarified butter, can also be used in cooking. Avoid sesame, sunflower and corn oils, which contain lectins that are damaging to the Type B digestive tract.

HIGHLY BENEFICIAL
Olive oil

NEUTRAL
Cod liver oil
Ghee
Linseed (flaxseed) oil

AVOID
Rapeseed oil
Corn oil
Cottonseed oil
Groundnut oil
Safflower oil
Sunflower oil
Sesame oil

Nuts and Seeds

BLOOD TYPE B		Weekly portion by ancestry		
Food	Portion	African	Caucasian	Asian
Nuts and seeds	Small handful	3–5x	2–5x	2–3x
Nut butters	15 g/½ oz	2–3x	2–3x	2–3x

Most nuts and seeds are not advised for Type Bs, so there is no highly beneficial category. Peanuts, sesame seeds and sunflower seeds, among others, contain lectins that interfere with Type B insulin production. It might be difficult for Type B Asians to give up sesame seeds and sesame-based products, but in this case, your blood type speaks more definitively than your culture.

NEUTRAL
Almonds
Almond butter
Brazil nuts
Chestnuts
Hickory nuts
Macadamia nuts
Walnuts

AVOID
Cashew nuts
Hazelnuts
Peanuts
Peanut butter
Pistachio nuts
Pine nuts
Poppy seeds
Sesame seeds
Sunflower margarine
Sunflower seeds
Tahini (sesame seed paste)

Beans and Pulses

BLOOD TYPE B		Weekly portion by ancestry		
Food	Portion	African	Caucasian	Asian
All recommended beans and pulses	60–90 g/2–3 oz (dry)	3–4x	2–3x	4–5x

Type Bs can eat some beans and pulses, but many beans, such as lentils, chick-peas, pinto beans and black-eye beans, contain lectins that interfere with the production of insulin.

Generally, Type B Asians tolerate beans and pulses better than other Type Bs because they are culturally accustomed to them. But even Asians should limit their selection of these foods to those that are highly beneficial, and eat them sparingly.

HIGHLY BENEFICIAL
Kidney beans
Lima beans
Navy beans

NEUTRAL
Broad beans
Cannellini beans
Green beans
Mangetouts
Peas – green, sugar-snap
Red soya beans

AVOID
Aduki beans
Black beans
Black-eyed beans
Chick-peas
Lentils – brown, green, red

Cereals

BLOOD TYPE B		Weekly portion by ancestry		
Food	Portion	African	Caucasian	Asian
All recommended cereals	115–175 g/4–6 oz (dry)	2–3x	2–4x	2–4x

When Type B is in good balance – that is, following the fundamental tenets of the diet – wheat may not be a problem. However, wheat is not tolerated well by most Type Bs. The wheat gluten contains a lectin that deposits in the muscle tissues, making them less efficient in burning calories and also depressing the metabolic rate. Foods that are not quickly metabolized are stored as fat, so wheat can be a factor in Type B weight gain.

Type Bs should also avoid rye, which contains a lectin that settles in the vascular system, causing blood disorders and the potential for strokes. (It is interesting to note that the main victims of vascular disease, sometimes called St Anthony's Fire, are the largely Type B population of Eastern European Jews. Rye bread is a popular part of their cultural tradition.)

Corn and buckwheat are also major factors in Type B weight gain. More than any other food, they contribute to a sluggish metabolism, insulin irregularity, fluid retention and fatigue.

Again, for Type Bs the key is balance. Eat a variety of grains and cereals. Rice and oats are excellent choices. I also urge you to try *spelt*, which is highly beneficial for Type Bs.

HIGHLY BENEFICIAL
Millet
Oat bran
Oatmeal
Rice bran
Rice – puffed
Spelt

NEUTRAL
Cream of rice
Familia
Farina
Granola
Grape nuts

AVOID
Amaranth
Barley
Buckwheat
Cornflakes
Cornmeal
Cream of wheat
Kamut
Rye
Shredded wheat
Wheat bran
Wheatgerm

Breads, Crispbreads and Muffins

BLOOD TYPE B   **Daily portion by ancestry**

Food	Portion	African	Caucasian	Asian
Breads, crispbreads	1 slice	0–1x	0–1x	0–1x
Muffins	1 muffin	0–1x	0–1x	0–1x

The recommendations here are similar to those for cereals. Avoid wheat, all corn products, buckwheat and rye. That still leaves a wide variety of breads to choose from. Try Essene bread, found in health food shops. These 'live' breads are highly nutritious. Although they are sprouted-wheat breads, the 'problem' kernel is destroyed in the sprouting process, and they are perfectly healthy.

HIGHLY BENEFICIAL
Brown rice bread
Fin crisps
Millet bread
Rice cakes
Sprouted-wheat Essence bread
Wasa bread

NEUTRAL
Gluten-free bread
Ideal flat bread
Oat bran muffins
Pumpernickel bread
Hi-protein bread
Spelt bread
Soya flour bread

AVOID
Bagels
Cornbread
Corn muffins
Durum wheat bread

Multi-grain bread
Polenta
100 per cent rye bread
Rye crisps
Ryvita crispbreads
Wheat bran muffins
Wholewheat bread

Grains and Pastas

BLOOD TYPE B   **Weekly portion by ancestry**

Food	Portion	African	Caucasian	Asian
Grains	200 g/7 oz (dry)	3–4x	3–4x	2–3x
Pastas	140–175 g/4–6 oz (dry)	3–4x	3–4x	2–3x

The Type B grain and pasta choices are absolutely consistent with the cereal and bread recommendations. I would, however, advise a moderated intake of pasta and rice. You won't need much of these nutrients if you're consuming the meat, seafood and dairy products advised.

HIGHLY BENEFICIAL
Oat flour
Rice flour

NEUTRAL
Graham flour
Plain flour
Quinoa – flour or grain
Rice – basmati, brown, white
Self-raising flour
Semolina pasta
Spelt flour
Spinach pasta

AVOID
Barley flour

Buckwheat flour
Bulgar wheat flour
Couscous
Durum wheat flour
Gluten flour
Rye flour
Soba (buckwheat) noodles
Tapioca
Wholewheat flour
Wild rice

Vegetables, Sprouts, Soya Products and Fresh Herbs

BLOOD TYPE B	Daily portion all ancestral types	
Food	Portion	
Raw	140–175 g/4–6 oz	3–5x
Cooked or steamed	140 g/5 oz	3–5x

There are many high-quality, nutritious, Type B-friendly vegetables – so take full advantage with three to five servings a day. There is only a handful of vegetables that Type Bs should avoid, but take these guidelines to heart.

Eliminate tomatoes completely from your diet. The tomato is classified as a rare vegetable called a *panhemaglutinan*. That means it contains lectin that can agglutinate every blood type. However, the tomato lectin has little effect on Type O or Type AB, while both Type B and Type A suffer strong reactions, usually in the form of irritations of the stomach lining.

Sweetcorn is also off the list as it contains those insulin and metabolism-upsetting lectins mentioned before. Also avoid olives, since their moulds can trigger allergic reactions.

Since Type Bs tend to be more vulnerable to viruses and autoimmune diseases, eat plenty of leafy green vegetables, which contain magnesium, an important anti-viral agent. Magnesium is also helpful for Type B children who have eczema.

For the most part, the vegetable world is your kingdom. Unlike other blood types, you can fully enjoy potatoes and yams, cabbages and mushrooms – and many other delicious foods from nature's bounty.

HIGHLY BENEFICIAL
Aubergines
Beetroots
Beetroot leaves
Broad beans
Brussels sprouts
Cabbage – chinese, red, white
Carrots
Cauliflower
Collard greens
Kale
Mushrooms – shiitake
Mustard greens
Parsley
Parsnips
Peppers – green, red, yellow
Sweet potatoes
Yams

NEUTRAL
Alfalfa sprouts
Asparagus
Bamboo shoots
Bok choy
Celery
Chervil
Chicory
Chilli peppers, jalapeño
Coriander
Courgettes
Cucumbers
Daikons
Dandelion greens

Dill
Endive
Escarole
Fennel
Garlic
Ginger
Horseradish
Jicama beans
Kohlrabi
Leeks
Lettuce – butterhead, Cos, iceberg, Webb
Mangetouts
Mesclun salad mixture
Mushrooms – abalone, chantarelles, cultivated, enoki, porcini, Portobello, tree oyster
Okra
Onions – green, red, Spanish, spring, yellow
Potatoes – red, white
Radicchio
Rappini
Rocket
Seaweeds
Shallots
Swedes
Spinach
Squash – all types
Swiss chard
Turnips
Water chestnuts
Watercress

AVOID
Avocado
Jerusalem artichokes
Globe artichokes
Mung bean sprouts
Olives – black, green, Greek, Spanish
Pumpkin

Radishes
Radish sprouts
Sweetcorn
Tempe
Tofu
Tomatoes

Fruits

BLOOD TYPE B	Daily portion – all ancestral types	
Food	**Portion**	
All recommended fruits	1 fruit or 90–140 g/3–5 oz	3–4x

There are very few fruits a Type B must avoid – and they're pretty uncommon in any case. Most Type Bs won't sorely miss persimmons, pomegranates or prickly pears in their diets.

Pineapple can be especially good for Type Bs who are susceptible to bloating – especially if they are not used to eating the dairy foods and meats on this diet. *Bromelain*, an enzyme in the pineapple, helps to digest food.

On the whole, choose fruits liberally from the following lists. Type Bs tend to have very balanced digestive systems, with a healthy acid–alkaline level, so they can enjoy fruits that are too acidic for other blood types.

Try to incorporate at least one or two fruits from the highly beneficial list every day to take advantage of their pro-B medicinal qualities.

HIGHLY BENEFICIAL
Bananas
Cranberries
Grapes – black, green, purple, red
Papaya
Pineapple
Plums – green, purple, red

NEUTRAL
Apples
Apricots
Blackberries
Blackcurrants
Blueberries
Boysenberries
Cherries
Dates
Elderberries
Figs – dried, fresh
Gooseberries
Grapefruit
Guava
Kiwi
Kumquats
Lemons
Limes
Loganberries
Lychees
Mangoes
Melons – canang, cantaloupe, casaba, Crenshaw, Christmas,
   honeydew, musk, Spanish
Nectarines
Oranges
Peaches
Pears
Plantains
Prunes
Raspberries
Redcurrants
Strawberries
Tangerines
Watermelons

AVOID
Coconuts
Persimmons

Pomegranates
Prickly pears
Rhubarb
Star fruit

Juices and Other Fluids

BLOOD TYPE B   Daily portion – all ancestral types

Food	Portion	
All recommended juices	225 ml/8 fl oz	2–3x
Water	225 ml/8 fl oz	4–7x

Most fruit and vegetable juices are okay for Type Bs. For a daily juice with built-in immune and nervous system boosters designed for Type Bs, try a **Membrane Fluidizer Cocktail** (I assure you that it's much more alluring than its name implies). Combine 1 tbsp flaxseed oil, 1 tbsp high-quality lecithin granules and 175–225 ml/6–8 fl oz fruit juice. Shake and drink.

Lecithin is a lipid, found in animals and plants, that contains metabolism- and immune system-enhancing properties. You can find lecithin granules in health food shops.

The **Membrane Fluidizer Cocktail** provides high levels of choline, serine and ethanolamine (the phospholipids), which are of great value to Type Bs. I find it tasty, because the lecithin emulsifies the oil, allowing it to mix with the juice.

HIGHLY BENEFICIAL
Cabbage juice
Cranberry juice
Grape juice
Papaya juice
Pineapple juice

NEUTRAL
Apple cider

Apple juice
Apricot juice
Black cherry juice
Carrot juice
Celery juice
Cucumber juice
Grapefruit juice
Orange juice
Other vegetable juices (*corresponding with highlighted vegetables on p. 163.*)
Prune juice
Water (with lemon juice)

AVOID
Tomato juice

Spices, Dried Herbs and Flavourings

Type Bs do best with warming spices, such as ginger, horseradish, curry powder and cayenne pepper. The exceptions are white and black pepper, which contain problem lectins. Avoid barley malt sweeteners, cornflour and cinnamon, as they tend to be stomach irritants. White and brown sugars, honey and molasses are sweet flavourings which respond in a neutral way to the Type B digestive system. Eat these sugars in moderation. Type Bs can also eat small quantities of chocolate, but consider it a condiment, not a main course!

HIGHLY BENEFICIAL
Curry powder
Horseradish
Parsley

NEUTRAL

Agar	Bergamot
Anise	Brown rice syrup
Arrowroot	Capers
Basil	Caraway seeds
Bay leaf	Cardamom

Carob
Cayenne pepper
Chervil
Chives
Chocolate
Coriander
Cream of tartar
Cumin
Dill
Garlic
Honey
Maple syrup
Marjoram
Mint
Miso
Molasses
Mustard – dry
Nutmeg
Paprika
Pepper – red flakes

Peppermint
Pimento
Rice syrup
Rosemary
Saffron
Sage
Salt
Savory
Seaweeds – dulse, kelp
Spearmint
Soy sauce
Sugar – brown, white
Tamarind
Tarragon
Thyme
Vanilla – essence, pod
Vinegars – balsamic, cider, herb,
    red and white wine, white

AVOID

Allspice
Almond essence
Barley malt
Cinnamon
Cornflour
Corn syrup

Gelatine – plain
Pepper – ground black and white,
    peppercorns

Condiments

Condiments are basically either neutral or bad for all types. Type
Bs can handle just about every common condiment, except
ketchup with its dangerous tomato lectins, but nutritional
common sense would suggest to limit your intake of foods that
provide no real benefit.

NEUTRAL
Jam (*from acceptable fruits on p. 165*)
Jelly (*from acceptable fruits on p. 165*)
Mayonnaise
Mustard
Pickles – dill, kosher, sweet, sour
Relish
Salad dressing (low-fat, from acceptable ingredients)
Worcestershire sauce

AVOID
Ketchup

Herbal Teas

Type Bs don't reap overwhelming benefits from most herbal teas, and only a few are harmful. Overall, Type Bs stay in balance with, for example, common sense teas – ginger to warm, peppermint to soothe the digestive tract and so on.

Ginseng is highly recommended for Type Bs because it seems to have a positive effect on the nervous system. Be aware, though, that it can act as a stimulant, so drink it early in the day.

Liquorice is particularly good for Type Bs. It has anti-viral properties that work to reduce susceptibility to autoimmune diseases. Also, many Type Bs experience a drop in blood sugar after meals (hypoglycaemia), and liquorice helps to regulate blood-sugar levels.

More recently, I've discovered that liquorice is a fairly powerful elixir for people suffering from ME/Chronic Fatigue Syndrome (See Chapter 9).

HIGHLY BENEFICIAL
Ginger
Ginseng
Liquorice
Liquorice root (with doctor's permission)
Parsley
Peppermint
Raspberry leaf

Rose-hip
Sage

NEUTRAL

Alfalfa	Hawthorn
Burdock root	Horehound
Catnip	Sarsaparilla
Cayenne	Spearmint
Camomile	St John's wort
Chickweed	Strawberry leaf
Dandelion	Thyme
Dong quai (Chinese angelica)	Valerian
Echinacea	Vervain
Elderflower	Yarrow
Green tea	Yellow dock

AVOID

Aloe
Coltsfoot
Cornsilk
Fenugreek
Gentian
Golden seal
Hops
Linden
Mullein
Red clover
Rhubarb
Senna
Shepherd's purse
Scullcap

Miscellaneous Beverages

Type Bs do best when they limit their beverages to herbal and green teas, water and juice. Although beverages like coffee, black tea and wine do no real harm, the goal of the blood type diet is to maximize your performance, not to keep it in neutral. Caffeinated coffee or tea drinkers should replace these beverages with green tea, which has caffeine but also provides some antioxidant benefits.

HIGHLY BENEFICIAL
Green tea

NEUTRAL
Coffee – decaffeinated, regular
Lager
Tea – decaffeinated, regular
Wine – red, white

AVOID
Distilled spirits
Soda – Cola, diet, others
Seltzer water

MEAL PLANNING FOR TYPE B

The following sample menus and recipes will give you an idea of a typical diet beneficial to Type Bs.

See pages 81–82 for the general introduction to meal planning.

As you become more familiar with the Type B Diet recommendations, you'll be able to easily create your own menu plans and adjust favourite recipes to make them Type B-friendly.

An asterisk (*) denotes the recipe follows – recipes may occur in more than one of the four diets; if so there will be a page reference.

* * *

STANDARD MENU	WEIGHT CONTROL ALTERNATIVES

Sample meal plan No. 1

Breakfast
Membrane Fluidizer Cocktail
(*optional – see p. 167*)
2 slices Essene bread *with*   1 slice Essene bread
*Yogurt-Herb Cheese
poached egg
green tea

Lunch
Greek Salad – chopped lettuce,
    cucumber, spring onions,
    celery with a sprinkling feta
    cheese, oil and lemon.
banana
iced herbal tea

Mid-afternoon snack   1 scoop of low-fat cottage
Quinoa Apple Sauce Cake (*see*   cheese with pear slices
recipe p. 90)
herbal tea

Dinner
Lamb and Asparagus Stew   grilled lamb chop
(*see recipe p. 86*)
*Saffron Brown Rice   steamed asparagus
steamed vegetables (broccoli,
    Chinese cabbage, etc.)
frozen yogurt
(wine if desired)

Sample meal plan No. 2

Breakfast
Membrane Fluidizer Cocktail
(*optional – see p. 167*)
rice bran cereal with banana and
    skimmed milk
grape juice
coffee

Lunch

thin slice of cheese (Swiss or munster) *with*	
1 thin slice of turkey breast	2 slices turkey breast
2 slices spelt bread with mustard or mayonnaise	1 slice spelt bread with mustard only
green salad	
herbal tea	

Mid-afternoon snack
fruit-juice-sweetened yogurt
herbal tea

Dinner
*Grilled Fish
steamed vegetables (from accept-
    able list)
*Roasted Yams with Rosemary
mixed fresh fruit (from accept-
    able list)
herbal tea or coffee
(red or white wine if desired)

Sample meal plan No. 3

Breakfast
Membrane Fluidizer Cocktail
(*optional – see p. 167*)
Maple Walnut Granola (*see*   puffed rice with goat's milk
   recipe p. 90) with goat's milk
1 soft-boiled egg
grapefruit juice
green tea

Lunch
Spinach Salad (*see recipe p. 89*)
tuna with mayonnaise   plain tuna
rice cakes (no limit)   Essene bread
herbal tea

Mid-afternoon snack
Apricot Fruit Bread (*see recipe*   low-fat yogurt with raisins
   p. 133)
apple
coffee or tea

Dinner
*Scrumptious Fettucine Alfredo
green salad
frozen yogurt
herbal tea
(red or white wine if desired)

RECIPES

Grilled Fish*

90 g/3 oz unsalted butter, ghee or oil
1 tsp Tabasco sauce
1 tbsp chopped garlic
4 slices of your favourite thick fish fillet, such as cod or halibut
140 g/5 oz puffed rice cereal, crushed
2 tbsp chopped fresh parsley

Preheat the grill to high. Melt the butter. Add the Tabasco sauce
and garlic and fry until the garlic browns. Pour 4 teaspoons into
an ovenproof dish. Arrange the fish in a single layer. Sprinkle
the crushed cereal and parsley over the fish. Add rest of the
butter mixture on top of the fish.

Grill for 10–15 minutes until the fish flakes easily when tested
with the tip of a knife. Serve immediately.

Serves 4

Scrumptious Fettuccine Alfredo

225 g/8 oz rice or spelt fettucine or linguine
1 tbsp extra virgin olive oil
75 ml/6 fl oz buttermilk
25 g/1 oz Parmesan cheese, grated
75 g/2³/₄ oz spring onions sliced
2 tbsp chopped fresh basil
¹/₄ tsp finely grated lemon rind
¹/₄ tsp garlic powder or freshly pressed garlic
Extra Parmesan Cheese and fresh basil, to garnish
Lemon wedges, to serve

Cook pasta in a pan of boiling salted water until *al dente*. Drain
and immediately return to pan. Add the olive oil and toss to coat
the pasta.

In same pan as pasta, combine buttermilk, Parmesan cheese,

*My patient and friend, Cheryl Miller, is a wonderful cook. She supplied this
recipe, and it's just delicious.

spring onions, basil, lemon rind and garlic. Cook everything together over a medium-high heat until bubbly, stirring constantly.

Garnish with extra Parmesan cheese and fresh basil. Serve with lemon.

Makes 4 side dishes

Roasted Yams With Rosemary

This is a wonderful dish to have with a green salad or other roasted vegetables.

50 ml/2 fl oz extra virgin olive oil
1 tbsp chopped fresh rosemary, or 2 tsp dried
Dash of cayenne pepper or Cajun spice
5–6 medium yams, quartered

Preheat the oven to 180–190° C/350–375 F/Mark 4–5. Blend the olive oil, rosemary and spice together and place in an ovenproof dish. Add the yams and bake for 1 hour.

Serves 4

Saffron Brown Rice

400 g/14 oz brown basmati rice
3 tbsp extra-virgin olive oil
1 large Spanish onion or red onion, finely chopped
1 tsp ground coriander
1 tsp grated nutmeg
seeds from 2 cardamom pods
1 tsp saffron threads
2 tbsp rosewater
4 cups filtered water, boiling

Rinse the rice in a sieve under running water until the water runs clear. Then place the rice in a bowl, cover with cold water and leave to soak for 30 minutes. Drain well.

Heat the oil and sauté onion with all spices for 10 minutes over a low heat. In a small dish, beat the saffron and add rosewater.

To the onion mixture, add 1 tablespoon of the rosewater

mixture. Simmer for another 15 minutes and then add the rice with the filtered boiling water. Return to the boil, then lower the heat, cover and simmer for 35–40 minutes until tender. Just before serving add the rest of the rosewater.

Serves 4

Yogurt-Herb Cheese

1.8 kg/4 lb virtually fat-free natural yogurt
2 garlic cloves, very finely chopped
1 tbsp olive oil
1 tsp fresh thyme
1 tsp chopped fresh basil
1 tsp fresh oregano
salt and pepper, to taste
raw vegetables from acceptable list, to serve

Spoon the yogurt into a piece of muslin, then tie the cloth into a ball with string and allow the yogurt to drip over the kitchen sink or a bathtub for $4\frac{1}{2}$–5 hours.

Remove yogurt from muslin and transfer to a bowl. Stir in the remaining ingredients. Cover and chill for 1–2 hours before serving.

Serves 4–6

TYPE B SUPPLEMENT ADVISORY

The role of supplements – be they vitamins, minerals or herbs – is to add the nutrients that are lacking in your diet, and to provide extra protection where you need it. The supplement focus for Type Bs is:

- Fine-tuning an already balanced diet
- Improving insulin production
- Strengthening viral immunity
- Improving brain clarity and focus

Type Bs are a special (you might say lucky) case. For the most part, they can avoid major diseases by following this blood type diet. Because the diet is so rich in vitamins A, B, C and E, plus minerals, calcium and iron, there is no need for supplementation of these. Enjoy your unique status – but follow the diet!

The following are the few supplements that can benefit Type Bs.

BENEFICIAL

Magnesium

While the other blood types risk calcium deficiency, Type Bs risk magnesium deficiency. That's because Type Bs are so efficient in assimilating calcium that they risk creating an imbalance between the levels of calcium and magnesium. If this occurs, they become more at risk from viruses (or otherwise lowered immunity), fatigue, depression and, potentially, nervous disorders. In these instances, a trial of magnesium supplementation (3–500 mg) should be considered. Also, many Type-B children are plagued with eczema, and magnesium supplementation can often be beneficial.

Any form of magnesium is fine, although more patients report a laxative effect with magnesium citrate than with the other forms. An excessive amount of magnesium could, at least theoretically, upset the body's calcium levels, so be sure that you also consume high-calcium foods, such as cultured dairy products. The key is balance!

Best magnesium-rich foods for Type Bs (*see acceptable lists on pp. 150–172*)
all recommended green vegetables
grains
beans and pulses

Herbs/Phytochemicals recommended for Type Bs

Liquorice (*Glycyrrhiza glabra*)

Liquorice is a plant widely used by herbalists around the world. It contains at least four benefits – as a treatment for stomach ulcers, as an anti-viral agent against the herpes virus, to treat chronic fatigue syndrome and to combat hypoglycaemia.

Liquorice is a plant to be respected: large doses in the wrong person can cause sodium retention and elevated blood pressure. Anyone who suffers from hypoglycaemia, a condition where the blood sugar drops after a meal, should drink a cup or two of liquorice tea after meals. For Chronic Fatigue Syndrome, I recommend liquorice preparations, other than DGL and liquorice tea, but only under the guidance of a GP. Liquorice freely used in its supplemental form can be toxic.

Digestive enzymes

Any Type B who is not used to eating meat or dairy foods may experience some initial difficulty adapting to the diet. Take a digestive enzyme with main meals for a while, and you'll adjust more readily to concentrated proteins. *Bromelain*, an enzyme found in pineapples, is available in supplemental form at health food shops, usually in the 4x strength.

Adaptogenic herbs

Adaptogenic herbs increase concentration and memory retention, sometimes a problem for Type Bs with nervous or viral disorders. The best are Siberian ginseng (*Eleutherococcus senticosus*) and *Gingko biloba*, both widely available from herbalists and health food shops. Siberian ginseng has been shown in Russian studies to increase the speed and accuracy of teletype operators.

Gingko biloba is currently the most frequently prescribed drug of any kind in Germany, where more than 5 million people take it daily. It increases the micro-circulation to the brain, which is why it is often prescribed to the elderly. It is currently being promoted as a brain stimulant, a pick-me-up for the mind.

Lecithin
Lecithin, a blood enhancer found principally in soya beans, allows the cell surface B antigens to move around more easily and better protect the immune system. Type Bs should seek this benefit from lecithin granules, not soya itself, as soya doesn't have the concentrated effect. Drinking the **Membrane Fluidizer Cocktail** (*see page 167*) is a good habit to develop, as it is a rather pleasant means of really stimulating your immune system.

TYPE B STRESS-EXERCISE PROFILE
The Type B response to stress represents a balance of the nervous mental activity of Type A and the more physically aggressive reactions of Type O. Type Bs temper each of these qualities and therefore respond with harmony and balance – harnessing the best qualities of the other blood types.

The Type B response to stress is an evolutionary sophistication demanded by a multidimensional environment. Human beings needed both the physical endurance required to conquer new lands, as well as the skills and patience to develop those lands. Remember, early Type Bs were represented by both barbarians and agrarians.

Type Bs confront stress very well for the most part, because they blend easily into unfamiliar situations. They are less confrontational than Type Os, but more physically charged than Type As.

Type Bs do well with exercises that are neither too aerobically intense nor completely aimed at mental relaxation. The ideal balance for many Type Bs is moderate activities that involve other people – like group hiking, biking excursions, the less aggressive martial arts, tennis and aerobics classes. You don't do as well when the sport is fiercely competitive – such as squash, football or basketball.

* * *

The most effective exercise schedule for Type Bs should be three days a week of intense physical activity, and two days a week of relaxation exercises.

Exercise	Duration (minutes)	Frequency – times per week
AEROBICS	45–60	3
TENNIS	45–60	3
MARTIAL ARTS	30–60	3
CALISTHENICS	30–45	3
HIKING	30–60	3
CYCLING	45–60	3
SWIMMING	30–45	3
BRISK WALKING	30–60	3
JOGGING	30–45	3
WEIGHT TRAINING	30–45	3
GOLF	60	2
T'AI CHI	45	2
HATHA YOGA	45	2

Type B Exercise Guidelines

FOR PHYSICAL EXERCISE:
The Guidelines here are exactly the same as for Type O – please refer to pp. 97–98.

FOR RELAXATION EXERCISE:
T'ai chi and yoga are the perfect way to balance the more physical activities of your week.

T'ai Chi
Tai chi ch'uan (or *t'ai chi*) is an exercise that enhances the flexibility of body movement. The slow, graceful, elegant gestures of the routines hardly resemble the original full-speed hand and foot blows, blocks and parries they represent. In China, *t'ai chi* is practised daily by groups who gather in parks and public squares to perform the movements in unison. *T'ai chi* can be a very effective relaxation technique, although it takes concentration and patience to master.

Yoga
The guidelines and simple relaxation techniques are the same as those for Type A – please refer to pp. 143–145.

TYPE B: THE PERSONALITY QUESTION

Early Type Bs, confronted with new lands, unfamiliar climates and the intermingling of races, had to be flexible and creative in order to survive. Type Bs required less ordered and harmonious conformity than the settled Type As, as well as less of the hunter's purposefulness that characterized Type Os.

These same characteristics exist in the very cells of Type Bs. Biologically, Type Bs are more flexible than Type Os, Type As or Type ABs – less vulnerable to many diseases common to the others. The Type B who lives in harmony – working, exercising and eating in a balanced way – is the essence of a survivor.

In many ways, Type Bs have the best of all possible worlds. They have elements of the mental, more sensitively agitated activity of the Type A, with the sheer physical reactions and aggression of the Type O. Perhaps Type Bs relate more easily to different personality types because they are genetically more in harmony and thus feel less inclined to challenge and confront. They can see others' points of view; they are empathic.

The Chinese, Japanese and many other Asian societies are composed of a high number of Type Bs. Chinese medicine – ancient, natural and complex – places a great emphasis on balancing the physiological and emotional states. Unbridled joy (a desirable state for most Westerners) is viewed by Chinese physicians as being dangerous to the balance of the heart. Balance and harmony is a very Type B kind of medicine.

Traditional Jewish populations are primarily Type B, regardless of their geographic locations. Jewish religion and culture represent the blending of mind, soul and matter. In Jewish tradition, intelligence, peace and spirituality live side-by-side with a forceful physicality and readiness for battle. To many people, this seems like a contradiction. It is really the harmonious energies of the Type B in action.

7
Blood Type AB Plan

TYPE AB: THE ENIGMA
- Modern merging of A and B
- Chameleon's response to changing environmental and dietary conditions
- Sensitive digestive tract
- Overly tolerant immune system
- Responds best to stress spiritually, with physical verve and creative energy
- An evolutionary mystery

Contents

THE TYPE AB DIET

Blood Type AB is less than a thousand years old, rare (2–5 per cent of the world's population), and biologically complex. It doesn't fit comfortably into any of the other categories. Multiple antigens make Type ABs sometimes A-like, sometimes B-like and sometimes a fusion of both – kind of a blood type centaur.

This multiplicity of qualities can be positive or negative, depending on the circumstances, so the Type AB diet requires careful reading of foods lists, and familiarization with both the Type A and Type B diets to better understand the parameters of this diet.

Essentially, most foods which are not recommended for either Type A or Type B are probably bad for Type AB, although there are some exceptions. *Panhemaglutinans*, which are lectins capable of agglutinating all of the blood types, seem to be better tolerated by Type ABs, perhaps because the lectin's reaction is diminished by the double A and B antibodies. Tomatoes are an excellent example: Type A and Type B cannot tolerate the lectins, while Type AB eats tomatoes with no discernible effect.

Type ABs are often stronger and more active than the more sedentary Type As. This extra dollop of *élan vital* may be because their genetic memories still contain remnants of their steppe-dwelling Type B ancestors.

The Weight Loss Factor

When it comes to gaining weight, Type ABs reflect the mixed inheritance of their A and B genes. Sometimes that means special problems. For example, Type ABs have Type A's low stomach acid, along with Type B's adaptation to meats. So, although they are genetically programmed for the consumption of meats, they lack enough stomach acid to metabolize them efficiently, and the meat that is eaten gets stored as fat. For weight loss, consumption of meats should be restricted, only eating small amounts that are supplemented with vegetables and tofu.

Type B propensities cause the same insulin reaction when dried kidney or lima beans, corn, buckwheat or sesame seeds are eaten, although the Type A side makes an AB friendly to lentils and peanuts. Inhibited insulin production causes hypoglycaemia, a lowering of blood sugar after meals, and leads to less efficient metabolism of foods.

Type ABs lack the severe reaction of Type Os and Type Bs to wheat gluten. But again, for weight loss purposes, they should avoid wheat, which tends to make muscle tissue more acidic. Type ABs utilize calories most efficiently when the tissue is somewhat alkaline.

Foods That Encourage Weight Gain

red meat	poorly digested; stored as fat

kidney beans lima beans seeds sweetcorn buckwheat	inhibit insulin production; cause hypoglycaemia

wheat	decreases metabolism inefficient use of calories

Foods That Encourage Weight Loss

tofu seafood green vegetables	promote metabolic efficiency

kelp dairy products	improve insulin production

alkaline fruits	increase muscle alkalinity

pineapple	aids digestion stimulates intestinal mobility

Incorporate these guidelines into the total picture of the Type AB diet that follows.

Meat, Offal, Poultry and Game

BLOOD TYPE AB   Weekly portion by ancestry

Food	Portion	African	Caucasian	Asian
Lean red meats, offal and game	115–175 g/4–6 oz (*men*) 60–140 g/2–5 oz (*women and children*)	1–3x	1–3x	1–3x
Poultry and feathered game	115–175 g/4–6 oz (*men*) 50–140 g/2–5 oz (*women and children*)	0–2x	0–2x	0–2x

*Remember: the portion recommendations of all food groups are merely guidelines that can help you refine your diet according to ancestral propensities.

When it comes to eating meat, offal, poultry and game, Type ABs borrow characteristics from both Type A and Type B. Similar to Type A, they do not produce enough stomach acid to effectively digest too much animal protein. Yet, the key is portion size and frequency. Type ABs need some animal protein, especially the kinds of meat that represent their B-like heritage – lamb, mutton, rabbit and turkey, instead of beef. The lectin that irritates the blood and digestive tracts of Type Bs has the same effect on Type ABs who should avoid eating chicken.

Also avoid all smoked or cured meats. These foods can cause stomach cancer in people with low levels of stomach acid, a trait ABs have in common with Type As.

HIGHLY BENEFICIAL
Lamb
Mutton
Rabbit
Turkey

NEUTRAL
Liver – calf, chicken, pig
Pheasant

AVOID
Bacon
Beef, including minced
Buffalo
Chicken
Duck
Goose
Ham
Heart
Partridge
Pork
Poussin
Veal
Venison
Quail

Seafood

BLOOD TYPE AB   **Weekly portion by ancestry**

Food	Portion	African	Caucasian	Asian
All seafood	115–175 g/4–6 oz	3–5x	3–5x	4–6x

There are a wide variety of seafoods for Type ABs and it is an excellent source of protein. Like Type As, ABs find it difficult to digest the lectins found in sole and plaice. Type ABs also share the Type A susceptibility to breast cancer. Anyone with Type AB blood with a family history of breast cancer should eat snails. The edible snail, *Helix pomatia*, contains a powerful lectin that specifically agglutinates mutated A-like cells for two of the most common forms of breast cancer. (See Chapter 10.) This is a positive kind of agglutination; the snail lectin gets rid of 'sick' cells.

HIGHLY BENEFICIAL

Albacore (tuna)   Red Snapper
Cod   Rainbow trout
Grouper   Sailfish
Hake   Sardines
Mackerel   Sea trout
Mahi mahi   Shad
Monkfish   Snails
Pike   Sturgeon
Porgy
Red fish

NEUTRAL

Abalone   Salmon
Bluefish   Scallops
Carp   Shark
Catfish   Smelts
Caviar   Snapper
Crockers   Squid
Herring – fresh,   Swordfish
Mussels

AVOID

Anchovy   Herring – pickled
Barracuda   Lobster
Clams   Octopus
Conch   Oysters
Crab   Plaice
Crayfish   Sea Bass
Eels   Shrimp
Frogs' legs   Smoked salmon
Haddock   Sole
Halibut   Striped bass

Dairy Products and Eggs

BLOOD TYPE AB   **Weekly portion by ancestry**

Food	Portion	African	Caucasian	Asian
Eggs	1 egg	3–5x	3–4x	2–3x
Cheeses	60 g/2 oz	2–3x	3–4x	3–4x
Yogurt	115–175 g/4–6 oz	2–3x	3–4x	1–3x
Milk	125–175 g/4–6 fl oz	1–6x	3–6x	2–5x

For dairy foods, Type ABs can put on the 'B' hat. Dairy products are beneficial, especially cultured and soured products – buttermilk, yogurt, kefir and reduced-fat sour cream – all of which are more easily digested.

The primary factor to watch out for is excessive mucus production. Like Type As, Type ABs already produce a lot of mucus, and don't need more. They should watch for signs of respiratory problems, sinus attacks or ear infections, that might indicate a need to cut back on the dairy foods.

Eggs are a very good source of protein for Type ABs. Although they're very high in cholesterol and Type ABs (like Type As) have some susceptibility to heart conditions, research indicates cholesterol-containing foods are not the real culprits, but, rather, saturated fats.

However, when eating eggs, increase the protein and lower the cholesterol intake by using two egg whites for every one egg yolk. (Note that the lectin found in the chicken muscle is not present in eggs.)

HIGHLY BENEFICIAL
Cottage cheese
Farmers cheese
Goat's cheese
Goat's milk
Kefir
Mozzarella cheese
Ricotta cheese

NEUTRAL
Cheddar cheese
Crème fraîche
Edam cheese
Emmenthal cheese
Fromage frais
Gouda cheese
Gruyère cheese
High-/low-fat soft cheese
Jarlsburg cheese
Milk – skimmed, semi-skimmed
Munster cheese
Neufachâtel cheese
Quark
Soya cheese*
Soya milk*
Whey
Yogurt – frozen, Greek-style, with fruit

Good dairy alternatives

AVOID
Blue cheese
Brie
Butter
Buttermilk
Camembert
Ice-cream
Parmesan cheese
Provolone cheese
Sherbet

Oils and Fats

BLOOD TYPE AB		Weekly portion by ancestry		
Food	Portion	African	Caucasian	Asian
Oils	1 tbsp	1–5x	4–8x	3–7x

Type ABs should use olive oil rather than animal fats (butter, lard), hydrogenated vegetable fats (margarine) or other vegetable oils. Olive oil is a mono-unsaturated fat which is believed to contribute to lowering blood cholesterol. They may also use small amounts of ghee, which is similar to clarified butter and used in Indian cooking.

HIGHLY BENEFICIAL
Olive oil

NEUTRAL
Rapeseed oil
Cod liver oil
Linseed (flaxseed) oil
Groundnut oil

AVOID
Corn oil
Cottonseed oil
Safflower oil
Sunflower oil
Sesame oil

Nuts and Seeds

BLOOD TYPE AB   **Weekly portion by ancestry**

Food	Portion	African	Caucasian	Asian
Nuts and seeds	Small handful	2–5x	2–5x	2–3x
Nut butters	15 g/½ oz	3–7x	3–7x	2–4x

Nuts and seeds present a mixed picture for Type ABs. They should be eaten in small amounts and with caution. Although nuts and seeds, and products made from them, can be a good supplementary protein source, all seeds contain the insulin-inhibiting lectins that make them a problem for Type Bs. On the other hand, ABs share the Type A preference for peanuts, which are powerful immune boosters.

Type ABs also tend to suffer from gall-bladder problems, so nut butters are preferable to whole nuts.

HIGHLY BENEFICIAL
Chestnuts
Peanuts
Peanut butter
Walnuts

NEUTRAL
Almonds
Almond butter
Brazil nuts
Cashew nuts
Hickory nuts
Macadamia nuts
Pine nuts
Pistachio nuts

AVOID
Hazelnuts
Poppy seeds
Pumpkin seeds
Sesame seeds
Sunflower margarine
Sunflower seeds
Tahini (sesame seed paste)

Beans and Pulses

BLOOD TYPE AB		Weekly portion by ancestry		
Food	Portion	African	Caucasian	Asian
All beans and pulses	60–90 g/2–3 oz (dry)	3–5x	2–3x	4–6x

Beans and pulses are another mixed bag for Type ABs. Lentils, navy and pinto beans are high-quality foods for Type ABs, although they are not advised for Type Bs. In particular, lentils are known to contain cancer-fighting antioxidants. On the other hand, dried kidney and lima beans, which slow insulin production in Type As, have the same effect in Type ABs.

HIGHLY BENEFICIAL
Lentils – green
Navy beans
Pinto beans
Red beans
Soya beans

NEUTRAL
Broad beans
Cannellini beans
Green beans
Green peas
Tamarind beans
Lentils – brown, red

AVOID
Aduki beans
Black beans
Black-eyed beans
Chick-peas
Kidney beans
Lima beans

Cereals

BLOOD TYPE AB		Weekly portion by ancestry		
Food	Portion	African	Caucasian	Asian
All recommended cereals	115–175 g/4–6 oz (dry)	2–3x	2–3x	2–4x

Guidelines for Type ABs favour both Type A and Type B recommendations. Generally, ABs do well on grains, even wheat, but must limit their wheat consumption because the inner kernel of the wheat grain is highly acid-forming for Type ABs. Wheat is also not advised if you are trying to lose weight. Type ABs with a pronounced mucus condition caused by asthma or frequent infections should also limit wheat consumption, as wheat causes mucus production. Experiment for yourself to determine how much wheat you can eat. Type ABs do best when their tissues are slightly alkaline. While the inner kernel of wheat grain is alkaline in Type Os and Type Bs, it becomes acidic in Type As and Type ABs.

Limit the intake of wheatgerm and bran to once a week. Oatmeal, soya flakes, millet, farina, ground rice and soya chunks and mince are good Type AB cereals, but ABs must avoid buckwheat and cornmeal.

HIGHLY BENEFICIAL
Millet
Oat bran
Oatmeal
Rice bran
Rice – puffed
Ryeberry
Spelt

NEUTRAL
Amaranth
Barley
Cream of rice
Cream of wheat
Familia
Farina
Granola
Wheatgerm
Shredded wheat
Wheat bran

AVOID
Buckwheat
Corn flakes

Cornmeal
Kamut

Breads, Crispbreads and Muffins

BLOOD TYPE AB **Daily portion by ancestry**

Food	Portion	African	Caucasian	Asian
Breads, crispbreads	1 slice	0–1x	0–1x	0–1x
Muffins	1 muffin	0–1x	0–1x	0–1x

The Type AB guidelines for eating breads and muffins are similar to cereals and grains. They are generally favourable foods, but are inadvisable for anyone who produces excessive mucus or is overweight. Soya and rice flour are good substitutes. Note that although Essene bread (found in health food shops) is sprouted-wheat bread, the gluten lectin is destroyed in the sprouting process. However, be aware that sprouted breads sold commercially often only contain a small proportion of sprouted wheat and are basically wholewheat breads. Read the ingredient labels. Avoid corn muffins and cornbread.

HIGHLY BENEFICIAL
Brown rice bread
Millet bread
Rice cakes
100 per cent rye bread
Rye crisps
Soya flour bread
Sprouted-wheat Essene bread
Ryvita crispbreads
Fin crisps
Wasa bread

NEUTRAL
Bagels
Durum wheat bread
Gluten-free bread

Ideal flat bread
Matzos
Multi-grain bread
Oat bran muffins
Pumpernickel bread
Hi-protein bread
Spelt bread
Wheat bran muffins
Whole-wheat bread

AVOID
Corn muffins
Cornbread
Polenta

Grains and Pastas

BLOOD TYPE AB		Weekly portion by ancestry		
Food	**Portion**	African	Caucasian	Asian
Grains	200 g/7 oz (dry)	2–3x	3–4x	3–4x
Pasta	140–175 g/4–6 oz (dry)	2–3x	3–4x	3–4x

Type ABs benefit from a diet rich in rice rather than pasta, although semolina or spinach pasta once or twice a week is fine. Again, avoid corn and buckwheat in favour of oats and rye. Limit eating bran and wheatgerm to once a week.

HIGHLY BENEFICIAL
Oat flour
Rye flour
Rice flour
Sprouted-wheat flour
Rice – basmati, brown, white
Wild rice

NEUTRAL
Couscous

Bulgar wheat flour
Durum wheat flour
Gluten flour
Graham flour
Plain flour
Quinoa – flour or grain
Self-raising flour
Semolina pasta
Spelt flour
White flour
Wholewheat flour

AVOID
Barley flour
Buckwheat flour
Soba (buckwheat) noodles
Tapioca

Vegetables, Sprouts, Soya Products and Fresh Herbs

BLOOD TYPE AB

Food	Portion	Daily portion – all ancestral types
Raw	140–175 g/4–6 oz (prepared)	3–5x
Cooked or steamed	140 g/5 oz (prepared)	3–5x

Fresh vegetables are an important source of phytochemicals, the natural substances in foods that have a tonic effect in cancer and heart disease prevention – diseases that afflict Type As and Type ABs more often as a result of weaker immune systems. These should be eaten several times a day. Type ABs have a wide selection – nearly all the vegetables that are good for either Type A or Type B are good for them as well.

The one exception is the *panhaemaglutinan* in tomatoes which affects all blood types. Since Type ABs have so much blood type material and the lectin isn't specific, they seem able to avoid the ill effects. I've tested Type ABs who were eating a lot of tomatoes, and their Indican Scales were clear.

Type ABs should make tofu a regular part of their diet, in combination with small amounts of meat and dairy products. Tofu also has well-acknowledged cancer-fighting benefits.

Like Type Bs, ABs must avoid fresh sweetcorn and all corn-based products.

HIGHLY BENEFICIAL
Alfalfa sprouts
Aubergines
Beetroots
Beetroot leaves
Broccoli
Cauliflower
Celery
Collard greens
Cucumbers
Dandelion greens
Garlic
Kale
Mushrooms – maitake
Mustard greens
Parsley
Parsnips
Sweet potatoes
Tempe
Tofu
Yams

NEUTRAL
Asparagus
Bamboo shoots
Bok choy
Brussels sprouts
Cabbage – Chinese, red, white

Carrots
Chervil
Chicory
Coriander
Courgettes
Daikons
Endive
Escarole
Fennel
Ginger
Horseradish
Jicama beans
Kohlrabi
Leeks
Lettuce – butterhead, Cos, iceberg, Webb
Mangetouts
Mesclun salad mixture
Mushrooms – abalone, chantarelles, cultivated, enoki, porcini,
   Portobello, shiitake, tree oysters
Okra
Olives – Greek, green, Spanish
Onions – Spanish, spring, red, yellow
Potatoes – red, white
Pumpkins
Radicchio
Rappini
Seaweeds
Shallots
Spinach
Squash – all types
Swedes
Swiss chard
Tomatoes
Turnips
Water chestnuts
Watercress

AVOID

Avocado
Broad beans
Chilli peppers, jalapeño
Globe artichokes
Jerusalem artichokes
Mung bean sprouts
Olives – black
Radishes
Peppers – green, red, yellow
Sweetcorn

Fruits

BLOOD TYPE AB	Daily portion – all ancestral types	
Food	Portion	
All recommended fruits	1 fruit or 90–140 g/3–5 oz	3–4x

Type ABs inherit mostly Type A intolerances and preferences for certain fruits. Focus on the more alkaline fruits, such as grapes, plums and berries, which can help to balance the grains that are acid-forming in muscle tissues.

Like Type As, Type ABs don't do well on certain tropical fruits, such as mangoes and guavas. But pineapple is an excellent digestive for Type ABs.

Oranges should also be avoided, even though they may well be favourites. Oranges are a stomach irritant for Type ABs, and they also interfere with the absorption of important minerals. To avoid confusion, let me reiterate once again that the acid/alkaline reaction happens two different ways – in the stomach and in the muscle tissues. Acidic oranges cause irritation in the sensitive, alkaline Type AB stomach. Although stomach acid is generally low in Type ABs, the acid contained in oranges irritates the delicate stomach lining. Grapefruit is closely related to oranges and is also an acidic fruit, but it has positive effects on the Type

AB stomach, exhibiting alkaline tendencies after digestion. Lemons are also excellent for Type ABs, helping to aid digestion and clear mucus from the system.

Since vitamin C is an important antioxidant, especially for stomach-cancer prevention, eat other vitamin C-rich fruits, such as grapefruit or kiwi.

The banana lectin interferes with Type AB digestion. I recommend substituting other high-potassium fruits such as apricots, figs and certain melons.

HIGHLY BENEFICIAL
Cherries
Cranberries
Figs – dried, fresh
Gooseberries
Grapes – black, green, purple, red
Loganberries
Plums – green, purple, red

NEUTRAL
Apples
Apricots
Blackberries
Blackcurrants
Blueberries
Boysenberries
Dates
Elderberries
Grapefruit
Kiwi
Kumquats
Lemons
Limes
Lychees
Melons – canang, cantaloupe, casaba, Crenshaw, Christmas, honeydew, musk, Spanish
Nectarines
Oranges

Papayas
Peaches
Pears
Pineapples
Plantains
Prunes
Raisins
Raspberries
Redcurrants
Strawberries
Tangerines
Watermelons

AVOID
Bananas
Coconuts
Guavas
Mangoes
Persimmons
Pomegranates
Prickly pears
Rhubarb
Star fruit

Juices and Other Fluids

BLOOD TYPE AB   Daily portion – all ancestral types

Food	Portion	
All recommended juices	225 ml/8 fl oz	2–3x
Water	225 ml/8 fl oz	4–7x

Type AB should begin each day by drinking a glass of warm water with the freshly squeezed juice of $\frac{1}{2}$ lemon to cleanse the system of mucus accumulated during sleep. The lemon water also aids elimination. Follow with a diluted glass of grapefruit of papaya juice. (As with other fruits, you may have to juice it yourself.)

Stress high-alkaline fruit juices like black cherry, cranberry or grape.

HIGHLY BENEFICIAL
Black cherry juice
Cabbage juice
Carrot juice
Celery juice
Cranberry juice
Grape juice
Papaya juice

NEUTRAL
Apple cider
Apple juice
Apricot juice
Cucumber juice
Grapefruit juice
Orange juice
Other vegetable juices (corresponding with highlighted vegetables on pp. 200–202.
Pineapple juice
Prune juice
Water (with lemon juice)

AVOID
Orange juice

Spices, Dried Herbs and Flavourings
Sea salt and kelp should be used in place of processed table salt. Their sodium content is comparatively low – a necessity for Type AB – and kelp has immensely positive heart and immune system benefits. It is also useful for weight control. Miso, made from soya beans, is very good for Type ABs, and makes a delicious soup or sauce.

Avoid all pepper and vinegar because they are acidic. Instead of vinegar, use lemon juice with oil and herbs to dress vegetables or salads. And don't be afraid to use generous amounts of garlic. It's a potent tonic and natural antibiotic, especially for Type ABs.

Sugar and chocolate are allowed in small amounts. Use them as you would condiments.

HIGHLY BENEFICIAL
Curry powder
Horseradish
Miso
Parsley

NEUTRAL

Agar
Arrowroot
Basil
Bay leaf
Bergamot
Brown rice syrup
Caraway seeds
Cardamom
Carob
Chervil
Chives
Chocolate
Cinnamon
Coriander
Cream of tartar
Cumin
Dill
Garlic
Honey
Maple syrup
Marjoram
Mint
Molasses

Mustard – dry
Nutmeg
Paprika
Peppermint
Pimento
Rice syrup
Rosemary
Saffron
Sage
Salt
Savory
Seaweeds – dulse, kelp
Soy sauce
Spearmint
Sugar – brown, white
Tamari
Tamarind
Tarragon
Thyme
Turmeric
Vanilla
Vinegars – balsamic, cider, red wine

AVOID
Allspice
Almond essence
Anise
Barley malt
Capers
Cayenne pepper
Cornflour
Corn syrup
Gelatine
Pepper – black or white peppercorns, ground, red pepper flakes
Tapioca
Vinegar, white

Condiments
Avoid all pickled condiments, due to a Type AB susceptibility to stomach cancer. Also avoid ketchup, which contains vinegar.

NEUTRAL
Jam (from acceptable fruits on pp. 203–204)
Jelly (from acceptable fruits on pp. 203–204)
Mayonnaise
Mustard
Salad dressing (low-fat, from acceptable ingredients)

AVOID
Ketchup
Pickles – dill, kosher, sweet, sour
Relish
Worcestershire sauce

Herbal Teas
Herbal tea should be drunk by Type ABs to rev up the immune system and build protections against cardiovascular disease and cancer. Alfalfa, aloe, burdock root, camomile and echinacea are immune-system boosters. Hawthorn and liquorice root are highly recommended for cardiovascular health. Green tea is very beneficial for the immune system. Dandelion, burdock root and strawberry leaf teas will aid absorption of iron and prevent anaemia. (You may need to infuse your own herbal teas.)

HIGHLY BENEFICIAL
Alfalfa
Burdock root
Echinacea
Ginseng
Ginger
Green tea
Hawthorn
Liquorice Root (with doctor's permission)
Rose-hip

NEUTRAL
Catnip
Cayenne
Camomile
Chickweed
Dandelion
Dong quai (Chinese angelica)
Elderflower
Golden seal
Horehound
Parsley
Peppermint
Raspberry leaf
Sage
Sarsaparilla
Spearmint
St John's wort
Strawberry leaf
Thyme
Valerian
Vervain
Yarrow
Yellow dock

AVOID
Aloe
Coltsfoot
Corn silk
Fenugreek
Gentian
Hops
Linden
Mullein
Red clover
Rhubarb
Senna
Shepherd's purse
Scullcap

Miscellaneous Beverages
Red wine is good for Type ABs because of its positive cardiovascular effects. A glass of red wine every day is believed to lower the risk of heart disease for both men and women.

A cup or two a day of regular or decaffeinated coffee increases stomach acid and also has the same enzymes found in soya beans. Alternate coffee and green tea for the best combination of benefits.

HIGHLY BENEFICIAL
Coffee – decaffeinated, regular
Green tea

NEUTRAL
Soda water
Lager
Seltzer water
Wine – red, white

AVOID
Distilled spirits
Tea – black, decaffeinated, regular
Soda – Cola, diet, others

MEAL PLANNING FOR TYPE AB
The following sample menus and recipes will give you an idea of a typical diet beneficial to Type ABs.

See pages 81–82 for the general introduction to meal planning.

As you become more familiar with the Type AB Diet recommendations, you'll be able to easily create your own menu plans and adjust favourite recipes to make them Type AB-friendly.

An asterisk (*) indicates the recipe follows – recipes may occur in more than one of the four diets; if so there will be a page reference.

* * *

STANDARD MENU	WEIGHT CONTROL ALTERNATIVES

Sample meal plan No. 1

Breakfast
water with juice ½ lemon (on rising)
diluted grapefruit juice
2 slices Essene bread — 1 slice Essene bread
Yogurt-Herb Cheese (*see recipe p. 178*) — 1 poached egg
decaffeinated coffee

Lunch
115 g/4 oz sliced turkey breast
2 slices rye bread — 1 slice rye bread or 2 rye crispbreads
Caesar salad
2 plums
herbal tea

Mid-afternoon snack
*Baked Tofu Cheesecake — 115 g/4 oz low-fat yogurt with fruit
iced herbal tea

Dinner
Tofu Omelettes (*see recipe p. 132*)
stir-fry vegetables (from acceptable list)
mixed fruit salad (from acceptable list)
decaffeinated coffee
(red wine if desired)

Sample meal plan No. 2

Breakfast
water with juice ½ lemon (on
  rising)
diluted grapefruit juice
Maple Walnut Granola (*see recipe
  p. 90*) with soya milk
decaffeinated coffee

Lunch
*Tabbouleh
bunch of grapes or apple
iced herbal tea

Mid-afternoon snack
Carob Chip Cookies (*see recipe   honeydew melon with 1 scoop
  p. 89*)   cottage cheese
coffee or herbal tea

Dinner
*Roasted Rabbit
Bean Salad (*see recipe p. 89*)
boiled basmati rice   steamed broccoli and
frozen yogurt   cauliflower
decaffeinated coffee
(red wine if desired)

Sample meal plan No. 3

Breakfast
water with juice ½ lemon (on
    rising)
diluted grapefruit juice
1 poached egg
2 slices essene bread *with*   1 slice Essene bread *with*
    organic almond butter   reduced-sugar jam
decaffeinated coffee

Lunch
Tofu-Pesto Lasagne (*see recipe*   tofu and vegetable stir-fry
    p. 131) *or*   (from acceptable list)
*Tofu-Sardine Fritters
mixed green salad
2 plums
herbal tea

Mid-afternoon snack
fruit-juice-sweetened yogurt

Dinner
grilled salmon with fresh dill and
    lemon
Saffron Brown Rice (*see recipe*   steamed asparagus
    p. 177)
Spinach Salad (*see recipe p. 89*)
decaffeinated coffee
(red wine if desired)

RECIPES

Baked Tofu Cheesecake*

700 g/1½ lb firm tofu, drained
150 ml/5 fl oz soya milk
¼ tsp salt (optional)
2 tsp lemon juice
finely grated rind of 1 lemon
1 tsp vanilla essence

For the pastry
90 g/3 oz wholemeal or rye flour
40 g/1½ oz rolled oats
½ tsp salt
125 ml/4 fl oz oil

To make the pastry, combine all the ingredients in a bowl with 2 tablespoons water and mix until the mixture holds together. Press over the base and side of a 20 cm/8 in loose-bottomed tin. Prick several times with a fork.

Meanwhile, preheat the oven to 150°C (300°F) Mark 2.

To make the filling, stir together the tofu, soya milk, salt, lemon juice and rind and vanilla. Pour into the prepared tin and level the surface. Bake for 35–40 minutes.

Makes approximately 8 slices

Roasted Rabbit

2 rabbits, cleaned, dressed and cut into serving pieces
225 ml/8 fl oz cider vinegar
1 small onion, chopped
115 g/4 oz rice flour or crushed wheat-free breadcrumbs
2 tsp salt
¼ tsp pepper
dash of ground cinnamon
75 g/2¾ oz margarine

---

*This recipe was given to me by Yvonne Chapman.

Marinate the rabbit pieces in a non-metallic bowl in the vinegar, onion, and half the salt for a few hours before cooking.

Meanwhile, preheat the oven to 190° C (375° F) Mark 5.

Combine the flour, remaining salt and spices in a plate.

Drain the rabbit pieces and pat dry. Dip rabbit in the melted margarine, then in flour or crushed breadcrumb mixture until well coated.

Place on a baking sheet and roast for 30–40 minutes

Serves 4–6

Tofu-Sardine Fritters*

1 can sardine fillets (deboned)
2 pieces, each 2.5 cm/1 inch, medium or firm tofu, drained
1/4 tsp horseradish powder
dash of cider vinegar
olive oil

Mash the sardines with a fork until fluffy. Mash the tofu into the sardines. Sprinkle in the horseradish powder, add a dash of vinegar and continue mixing ingredients until well blended.

Form the mixture into small patties. Heat a small amount of olive oil in a heavy-based frying pan. Brown both sides of patties, then drain well on kitchen paper. Alternatively, brown under a grill. Serve with a salad.

Serves 2

Tabbouleh

This makes a refreshing first course or picnic salad.

175 g/6 oz millet, cooked
1 bunch spring onions, chopped
1 large cucumber, peeled and chopped (optional)
4 bunches fresh parsley, chopped
1 bunch fresh mint, chopped
65 ml/2 1/2 fl oz olive oil
juice of three lemons

*Another recipe given to me by Yvonne Chapman.

1 tbsp salt
lettuce leaves, to serve

Place the millet in a large bowl. Add all chopped vegetables and herbs and mix well. Add oil, lemon juice and salt. Serve on a bed of lettuce leaves. Makes a refreshing appetizer or a picnic salad

Serves 4

TYPE AB SUPPLEMENT ADVISORY

The role of supplements – be they vitamins, minerals or herbs – is to add the nutrients that are lacking in your diet, and to provide extra protection where you need it. The supplement focus for Type ABs is:

- Supercharging the immune system
- Supplying cancer-fighting antioxidants
- Strengthening the heart

Type ABs present a somewhat mixed picture when it comes to supplements. Although ABs share the vulnerable immune system and disease susceptibilities of Type As, the Type AB diet provides a rich variety of nutrients with which to fight back.

For example, Type ABs get plenty of vitamin A, vitamin B12, niacin and vitamin E in their diets, supplying a dietary protection against cancer and heart disease. I would only suggest further supplementation if for some reason a Type AB isn't adhering to the diet. Even iron, which is seriously lacking in the Type A vegetarian diet, is readily available in Type AB foods. There are, however, some supplements that can be of benefit to Type ABs.

BENEFICIAL

Vitamin C

Type ABs – who have higher rates of stomach cancer because of low stomach acid – can benefit from taking additional supplements of vitamin C. For example, nitrate, a compound that results from the smoking and curing of meats, could be a particular problem with Type ABs, because its cancer-causing potential is greater in people with lower levels of stomach acid. As an antioxidant, vitamin C is known to block this reaction (although you should still avoid smoked and cured foods). However, don't take this to mean that massive amounts should be consumed. I have found that Type ABs do not do as well on high doses (1000 mg+) of vitamin C because it tends to upset their stomachs. Taken over the course of a day, two to four capsules of a 250 mg supplement, preferably derived from rose-hips, should cause no digestive problems.

Best C-rich foods for Type ABs
berries
broccoli
cherries
grapefruit
lemon
pineapple

Zinc (*with caution*)
I have found that a small amount of zinc supplementation (as little as 3 mg per day) often makes a big difference in protecting Type AB children against infections, especially ear infections. Zinc supplementation is a double-edged sword, however. While small, periodic doses enhance immunity, long-term, higher doses depress it and can interfere with the absorption of other minerals. Be careful with zinc! It's completely unregulated and is widely available as a supplement, but you really shouldn't use it without a GP's advice.

Best zinc-rich foods for Type ABs:
recommended meats (especially dark turkey meat)
eggs
beans and pulses

Selenium (*with caution*)
Selenium may be of value to Type ABs, as it seems to act as a component of the body's own antioxidant defences. However, cases of selenium toxicity have been reported in people who have taken excessive supplements. Check with your GP before taking this mineral.

Herbs/Phytochemicals recommended for Type ABs

Hawthorn (*Crataegus oxyacantha*)

With a tendency towards heart disease, Type ABs will want to be serious about protecting their cardiovascular system. Following the Type AB diet will have this effect, but anyone with a family history of heart disease or hardening of the arteries may want to take the preventive programme a step further. A phytochemical with exceptional preventive capacities is found in the hawthorn tree.

Hawthorn has a number of impressive antioxidant effects: it increases the elasticity of the arteries and strengthens the heart, while also lowering blood pressure and exerting a mild solvent-like effect upon the plaques in arteries. Officially approved for pharmaceutical use in Germany, the actions of hawthorn are virtually unknown elsewhere. Extracts and tinctures should be readily available through homeopathic GPs, health food shops and pharmacies. I cannot praise this herb too highly. Official German government monographs show the plant to be completely free of any side-effects. If I had my way, extracts of hawthorn would be used to fortify breakfast cereals, just like vitamins.

Immune-enhancing herbs

Because the immune systems of Type AB tend to be vulnerable to viruses and infections, gentle immune-enhancing herbs such as purple coneflower (*Echinacea purpurea*), can help to ward off colds or flus and may help optimize the immune system's anti-cancer surveillance. The Chinese herb huangki (*Astragalus membranaceous*) is also taken as an immune tonic. In both herbs the active ingredients are sugars that act as mitogens to stimulate white blood cell proliferation. The white blood cells, you will remember, defend the immune system.

Calming herbs

Type ABs can use mild herbal relaxants, such as camomile and valerian root. These herbs are available as teas and should be drunk frequently. Valerian has a bit of a pungent odour, which actually becomes pleasing once you get used to it.

Quercetin
Quercetin is a bioflavonoid found abundantly in vegetables, particularly yellow onions. Quercetin supplements are available in health food shops. It is a very powerful antioxidant, many hundreds of times more powerful than vitamin E. Quercetin makes a powerful addition to your cancer-prevention strategies.

Milk Thistle (*Silybum marianum*)
Like quercetin, milk thistle is an effective antioxidant with the additional special property of reaching very high concentrations in the liver and bile ducts. Type ABs tend to suffer from digestive disorders, particularly of the liver and gall-bladder. If there is any family history of liver, pancreas or gall-bladder problems, a milk thistle supplement should be taken. Cancer patients who are receiving chemotherapy should consult their GP about taking a milk thistle supplement to help protect their livers from damage. It is found in most health food shops.

Bromelain (*Pineapple enzymes*)
Type ABs suffering from bloating or other signs of poor absorption of protein should take a bromelain supplement. This enzyme, found in pineapples, has a moderate ability to break down dietary proteins, helping the Type AB digestive tracts more effectively assimilate proteins.

TYPE AB STRESS-EXERCISE PROFILE
The ability to reverse the negative effects of stress lives in your blood type. As discussed in Chapter 3, stress is not in itself a problem; it's how you respond to stress. Type ABs have inherited the exact stress pattern of Type As, and are not at all B-like.

Refer to pp. 141–142 as the stress/exercise profile is exactly the same as for Type A.

* * *

The following exercises are recommended for Type ABs. Pay special attention to the length of the sessions. To achieve a consistent release of tension and revival of energy it is necessary to perform one or more of these exercises three or four times a week.

Exercise	Duration (minutes)	Frequency – times per week
T'AI CHI	30–45	3–5
HATHA YOGA	30	3–5
AIKIDO	60	2–3
GOLF	60	2–3
CYCLING	60	2–3
BRISK WALKING	20–40	2–3
SWIMMING	30	3–4
DANCE	30–45	2–3
AEROBICS (low impact)	30–45	2–3
HIKING	45–60	2–3
STRETCHING	15	Every time you exercise

Type AB Exercise Guidelines
Follow the *Tai chi ch'uan* (or *t'ai chi*) and yoga guidelines on pp. 143–145.

TYPE AB: THE PERSONALITY QUESTION

Type AB followers of blood type-personality analysis love to boast that Jesus Christ was Type AB. Their evidence comes from blood tests conducted on the Shroud of Turin. It's a provocative idea, although I have my doubts since Jesus was supposed to have lived a good one thousand years before the emergence of Type AB.

But that's Type AB for you. They don't sweat about the details. Type AB is a merging of the edgy, sensitive Type A with the more balanced and centred Type B. The result is a spiritual, somewhat flaky nature that embraces all aspects of life without being particularly aware of the consequences. These characteristics are clearly evident in Type AB blood. The Type AB immune system is the best friend to nearly every virus and disease on the planet. If Type O has high-tech security gates on its immune system, Type AB doesn't even have a lock on its door.

Naturally, these qualities make Type ABs very appealing and popular. It's easy to like someone who welcomes you with open arms, doesn't hold grudges when you disappoint them and always says the most diplomatic thing in every situation. Not surprisingly, there are many healers and spiritual teachers who are Type AB.

The problem is, since Type ABs' immune systems are so indiscriminate, you begin to suspect that they have no loyalty to any one group.

On the positive side, Type ABs are considered to be members of one of the most captivating and interesting of the blood types. But their natural charisma can often lead to heartache. John F. Kennedy and Marilyn Monroe were both Type ABs, whose charisma exacted a heavy toll, but who both remain hauntingly prominent in public memory.

PART THREE

YOUR BLOOD TYPE
HEALTH

8
Medical Strategies:
The Blood Type Connection

BY NOW YOU are aware of the strong link between your blood type and your health. I hope you are also beginning to see that you can exert meaningful control, even when you have a susceptibility to a certain condition. Your Blood Type Plan is the cornerstone of a lifetime of good health.

In the next three chapters, I will talk in more detail about the specific medical issues that concern everyone, and how you can use your blood type information to make the best choices for your health. We begin with the drugs and treatments that are commonplace in modern life.

Drugs have been used as medicine for thousands of years. When a shaman, or witch doctor, brewed a potion, that potion had not only medical authority, but spiritual power. Although the infusion was often malodorous and vile, it contained magic, and the patient would gladly drink the bitter brew in hope of a cure.

Not that much has changed.

Today GPs over-prescribe medications, and we overuse them. It's a serious problem. Yet, unlike other naturopaths who reject the entire modern pharmacopoeia, I believe we must take a more reasoned and flexible point of view. Most medical preparations are designed to be effective on a broad range of the population, and should be used to treat the most severe and potentially dangerous conditions.

But let us also keep medication in perspective: all drugs are poisons. The good drugs that man has discovered over the centuries are selective poisons. Many others are broader, less-selective poisons. An excellent example of the latter is the diffuse arsenal of drugs used by oncologists for chemotherapy. In the process of destroying cancerous cells, many of these drugs indiscriminately attack healthy cells as well. The good news is that chemotherapy sometimes works, but the bad is that the patient sometimes dies of complications related to the treatment. It's a terrible conundrum.

Modern science has presented the medical community with a bewildering array of medications that are being prescribed worldwide by well-meaning doctors. But have we been careful enough in our use of antibiotics and vaccines? How do you know which medications are best for you, for your family, for your children?

Again, blood type holds the answer.

OVER-THE-COUNTER MEDICATIONS

There is a wide range of over-the-counter (OTC) medications designed for every common ailment – from headaches to aching joints to congestion to indigestion. On the face of it, these seem to be inexpensive, convenient, and effective remedies.

As a naturopathic physician, I try to avoid prescribing OTC medications whenever I can. In most cases, there are natural alternatives that work just as well or better. In addition, there are dangers inherent in using many OTC preparations, including:

- Aspirin's blood-thinning properties can be trouble for Type Os, who already have thin blood. Furthermore, they can mask the symptoms of a serious infection or illness.
- Antihistamines can raise blood pressure – a particular danger for Types A and AB. They can also cause sleeplessness and exacerbate prostate problems.
- Habitual use of laxatives actually can cause constipation, disrupting the natural process of elimination. They also can be harmful for people with Crohn's disease – primarily a Type O problem.
- Cough, throat, and chest remedies often have side effects, including high blood pressure, drowsiness, and dizziness.

Before you take an OTC remedy to treat a headache, cramps, or any other malady, investigate the possible causes of your problem. Often, it relates to your diet or stress. For example, you might ask:

- Is my headache a result of stress?
- Is my stomach discomfort caused by eating foods that are indigestible for my blood type?
- Are my sinus problems the result of mucus caused by eating too many mucus-generating foods? Or by eating histamine-releasing foods (such as wheat for Type O)?
- Is my flu virus the result of immune-system weaknesses?
- Is my congestion or bronchitis caused by an overproduction of mucus in my respiratory passages?
- Is my toothache caused by an infection that requires immediate medical treatment?
- Is my overreliance on commercial laxatives interfering with natural elimination and causing diarrhoea?

I urge you to seek medical attention if your symptoms are chronic or particularly severe. Pain, weakness, coughs, fever, congestion, and diarrhoea all can be signs of deeper problems. You might cover them up with medications, but you won't be addressing the root cause.

For occasional aches, pains and irregularities, the following remedies are excellent natural replacements for OTC drugs. They're available in many forms from your local health food shop or natural nutrition centre – including teas, compresses, liquid tinctures, extracts, powders, and capsules.

To make your own herbal tea, boil water and steep the natural herbs for about five minutes.

Please note the key indicating special considerations for each blood type.

Key

●	TYPE O AVOID
■	TYPE A AVOID
▼	TYPE B AVOID

†   TYPE AB AVOID

★   SPECIAL NOTE FOR ALL BLOOD TYPES

Headache
camomile
damiana ●
feverfew
valerian
white willow bark (*salix*)

Sinusitus
fenugreek ▼ †
thyme

Arthritis
alfalfa ●
boswella
calcium
epsom salt bath
rosemary tea soak

Earache
garlic-mullein-olive oil ear drops

Toothache
crushed garlic gum massage
oil of cloves gum massage

Indigestion, Heartburn
bladderwrack
bromelain (from pineapple)
gentian ● †
ginger
golden seal
peppermint

Cramps, Gas
camomile tea

fennel tea
ginger
peppermint tea
probiotic supplement with bifidus factor

Nausea
cayenne ■
ginger
liquorice root tea

Flu
arabino galacton
echinacea
garlic
golden seal
rose-hip tea

Fever
catnip ■
feverfew
vervain
white willow bark

Cough
coltsfoot ● ▼
horehound
linden ▼

Sore throat
fenugreek tea gargle ▼
golden seal root and sage tea gargle
stone root

Congestion
liquorice tea
mullein ▼
nettle
vervain

Constipation
aloe vera juice ● ▼ †
fibre ★ ★
larch tree bark (ARA-6) ★
psyllium
slippery elm

Diarrhoea
blueberries
elderberries
L. acidophilus (yogurt culture)
raspberry leaf

Menstrual cramps
Jamaican dogwood

★　　Currently under patent, substance of larch tree bark in a powdered form is available from my office under the name ARA-6. It has been tested to be an excellent natural immune system booster. Furthermore, a substance in larch tree bark, called butyrate, is a safe and effective natural source of fibre for all blood types. For more information and orders, see Appendix D.

★ ★　Natural fibre is available in many fruits, vegetables, and grains. Be sure to check your blood type food list before you choose a fibre source.

* * *

VACCINES: THE BLOOD TYPE SENSITIVITIES

Vaccination is an emotionally charged issue in both the conventional and alternative medical communities. From the more orthodox viewpoint, vaccination represents the first line of defence in preventive medicine. What are the consequences of placing increased emphasis on mandatory vaccination?

Vaccines have been of unquestioned benefit to mankind, saving hundreds of thousands of lives and preventing needless suffering. In the rare circumstances where there have been problems, the vaccines have sometimes reacted badly with a particularly hypersensitive individual. Our knowledge of the immune system does not yet reveal if vaccines have more profound resonances, possibly lowering some of our innate immunities to cancer. Yet, many public health officials and medical scientists behave as though it is somehow unpatriotic to question whether every new vaccine must be injected into the collective national bloodstream.

Meanwhile, the public remains confused. Parents want to know which vaccines, if any, their children should be exposed to. The elderly, the hypersensitive, and the pregnant worry about the effects of vaccinations. It shouldn't surprise you that there is no single answer for everyone. Your reaction to vaccines has a lot to do with your blood type.

Type O vaccine sensitivities

With all vaccines, parents of Type O children should be alert to any sign of inflammation, such as fever or joint pain, since the Type O immune system is prone to these reactions.

Avoid the injectable form of polio vaccine for Type O children, and opt instead for the oral preparation. Since Type Os have hyperactive immune systems, they do best with a less potent form of the vaccine.

Recently vaccinated Type O children should be carefully watched for a couple of days to insure that there are no complications. Don't give them acetaminophen, the most commonly prescribed OTC medication for vaccination-related problems. In my experience, Type O children seem to react poorly to this drug. Feverfew (*Tanacetum parthenium*), a herb which will work for Type Os, is available at most health food shops. Derived from the common chrysanthemum flower, in liquid tincture form, it can be given to a child every few hours. Four to eight drops of the tincture in a glass of juice is sufficient to achieve a positive effect.

If you are a pregnant woman with Type O blood, the flu vaccine holds special dangers, especially if the father of your baby is a Type A or Type AB. The flu vaccine could boost the presence of anti-A antibodies in your system, which could attack and damage your foetus.

Type A and Type AB vaccine sensitivities

Type A and Type AB children respond well to vaccines. A full vaccination programme – including the whooping cough vaccine – should produce few side-effects.

In contrast to Type O, Type A and Type AB children should take the injectable form of the polio vaccine because their digestive mucus does not react well to the oral polio vaccine.

Type B vaccine sensitivities

Type B children sometimes have severe neurological reactions to vaccinations. Parents should be acutely aware of any signal indicating complication, be it an alteration in your child's walking or crawling gait, or a personality change of some kind. If you intend to vaccinate your Type B child, it is imperative that you make sure he or she is first completely healthy – free of colds, flu or ear infections. Like Type Os, Type B children should use the oral form of polio vaccine.

Why do Type Bs tend to react so badly to vaccines? Type Bs produce an enormous number of B antigens in their nervous systems. I believe a cross-relation occurs in the Type B immune system when a vaccine is introduced that causes the body to turn and attack its own tissues. It may be the vaccine itself which causes this cross-reaction. Or perhaps it's one of the chemicals used to enhance the vaccine's effectiveness. It might even be the culture medium used to grow the vaccine. We just don't know yet.

Pregnant Type B women should also avoid the flu vaccine, especially if the father has Type A or Type AB blood. The flu vaccine could increase the production of anti-A antibodies, which could interfere with the healthy development of the foetus.

THE PROS AND CONS OF ANTIBIOTIC THERAPY

If your GP often prescribes antibiotics for simple colds and flu, I have one piece of advice: find another doctor.

The constant misuse of antibiotics is a leading factor in our growing inability to eradicate disease. The overuse of such wonder drugs promotes the development of progressively more resistant pathogens, which require ever stronger antibiotics for treatment. Far more powerful than any of the antibiotics currently being manufactured is the natural prescription of proper diet, proper rest and stress reduction.

Typically, there is a lag between the time you develop an infection and the time your body's immune system responds. It's like dialing 999; you know they aren't going to be at your door the second they answer your call. Antibiotics may get to an infection faster, but they hang up the phone on your body's own 999 emergency number – the immune system. Antibiotics basically cut off immune response; the body's responsibility for fighting an infection has been taken over by medication.

We race to treat fever with antibiotics, yet fever is generally a good sign. It indicates that the body's metabolic rate has kicked into overdrive, burning out invaders by making the environment as inhospitable to infectious organisms as it possibly can.

In my own practice I have discovered that the majority of people can eliminate an infection without the use of an antibiotic. Did you know that antibiotics only reduce the level of infection? Your body's immune system is still required to finish the battle. When you allow your body to go to war on its own terms, without antibiotic intervention, it develops not only a memory of specific antibodies to the current infection and any similar to it, but also the ability to fight more effectively the next time it is challenged or attacked.

A number of people are allergic to various antibiotics, but as a rule they produce few serious medical conditions. Very often, however, continued and heavy use of antibiotics destroys not only the infection, but all of the 'good' bacteria in the digestive tract. Many people experience diarrhoea, and quite often women become subject to recurring and persistent yeast infections, such as thrush. Supplements of a friendly digestive bacteria, *L. acidophilus*, may be taken in either tablet form or yogurt to restore the proper balance of bacteria in the digestive tract. (Both forms are available from health food shops.)

There are, of course, times when an appropriate antibiotic is needed and should be used. If you are given an antibiotic, take a supplement of bromelain to insure that your antibiotic spreads rapidly and penetrates tissue more readily. Pineapples contain this enzyme, so you may drink pineapple juice or take bromelain tablets when you're on a course of antibiotics.

Parents of sick children on antibiotics should set the alarm clock for 3 or 4 a.m. to administer an extra dose during the child's sleep cycle. This ensures a more rapid concentration of the drug to fight the infection.

Once more: if you need antibiotics, take them. If an infection becomes protracted, you certainly should consider using an antibiotic. I just think the body's immune system should be allowed to do what it's been created for – to resist.

Type O Antibiotic Sensitivities

Type Os should avoid penicillin-class antibiotics. The Type O immune system is more allergically sensitive to this class of drugs.

Also avoid sulpha-class drugs such as co-trimoxazole. They can cause skin rashes in Type Os.

Try to avoid macrolide-class antibiotics. Erythromycin and the newer macrolides such as azithromycin, can aggravate bleeding tendencies in Type Os. Be especially wary of this problem if you are currently taking blood-thinning medications such as warfarin.

Type A Antibiotic Sensitivities

Carbecephem-class antibiotics seem to work well for Type As. There are very few side-effects. Most Type As also respond well to penicillin-class and sulpha-class antibiotics. These are preferable to tetracycline or the newer macrolide-class antibiotics.

If a macrolide-class antibiotic is prescribed for a Type A, erythromycin is preferred over azithromycin. Both of these antibiotics can cause digestive problems and interfere with iron metabolism in the Type A system.

Type AB and Type B Antibiotic Sensitivities

Avoid quinolone-class antibiotics such as ciprofloxacin, if you can. If you must use them, take them in smaller doses than prescribed. Be aware of any sign of a nervous system disorder when taking a course of antibiotics, such as blurred vision, confusion, dizziness, or insomnia. Type AB and Type B should immediately discontinue the use of such medication and contact their GP.

ANTIBIOTIC THERAPY AT THE DENTIST
It is standard practice for dentists to use antibiotics as a preventive measure against infection. Patients with mitral valve prolapse, a heart condition, are always given a course of antibiotics to guard against any possibility of bacterial infection and subsequent valve damage.

However, a recent study in the *Lancet* found no benefit to a course of antibiotics for the majority of patients prior to invasive dental procedures. However, if you are a non-secretor, you run a much greater risk of infections following dental surgery than a secretor. There are many more instances of streptococcal bacteria causing endocarditis (an inflammation of the lining of the heart muscle) and rheumatic fever in non-secretors, because they produce much lower levels of protective antibodies in the mucous membranes of the mouth and throat. Secretors, on the other hand, have higher levels of these IgA antibodies which trap bacteria and destroy them before they can gain access to the bloodstream.

Non-secretors should always undertake preventive antibiotic therapy prior to any invasive dental procedure – from deep cleaning to oral surgery.

If you are Type O you may wish to opt out of antibiotic therapy, unless there is deep-rooted infection or the probability of heavy bleeding. Instead, try herbal medications with anti-strep activity, such as golden seal (*Hydrastis canadensis*).

Type A, Type B and Type AB may wish to discuss alternative therapies with their dentist or GP if they respond poorly to antibiotics.

Many dentists will refuse to treat a patient who declines the prophylactic use of antibiotics. If you are a healthy individual with no prior history of infections, consider going elsewhere for your dental work.

SURGERY: BETTER RECOVERY

Any invasive procedure is a shock to your system. Never take it lightly, even if it is a minor type of surgery. Boost your immune system in advance, no matter what your blood type.

Vitamins A and C have a profound effect on wound healing and minimize the formation of scar tissue. Every blood type can benefit from supplementation before surgery. Start taking vitamins A and C at least four days prior to surgery, and continue for at least a week afterwards. Every patient of mine who has followed this recommendation reports that both they and their surgeons were astonished at the rapidity of their recovery.

RECOMMENDED SURGICAL SUPPLEMENTATION PROTOCOL

Blood Type	Daily vitamin C	Daily vitamin A
Type O	2000 mg	30,000 IU
Type A	500 mg	10,000 IU
Type B Type AB	1000 mg	20,000 IU

Type O Surgical Cautions

Type Os often experience greater blood loss than other blood types during and after surgery because they have lower levels of serum-clotting factors. Make sure that you have plenty of vitamin K in your system before surgery; it is essential to clot formation. Kale, spinach and collard greens contain ample amounts of this vitamin, although you might want to supplement your diet with liquid chlorophyll. Chlorophyll supplements are available at health food shops.

Type Os with a history of phlebitis, or who are on a course of blood thinners, should consult their GP about supplementation recommendations. (It's worth noting that the thinner blood of Type Os does not necessarily protect against blood clots. Phlebitis often starts as an inflammatory condition of the veins that affects blood flow.)

Type Os can also boost their immune systems and metabolism with strong physical activity. If it is realistic for you to pursue this prior to surgery, exercise will allow your body to deal with the stress of surgery much more effectively, and also heal more rapidly.

Type B Surgical Cautions

Type Bs are fortunate in that they are less likely to experience post-surgical complications but the above vitamin protocol should be followed.

Type Bs who are suffering from a weakened condition may also want to use a couple of immune-boosting herbal teas prior to surgery. Burdock root (*Arctium lappa*) and purple coneflower (*Echinacea purpurea*) are excellent immune boosters. A few cups of tea taken every day over a number of weeks can be a positive stimulant for your immune system.

Type A and Type AB Surgical Cautions

Type A and Type AB are both more prone to post-surgical bacterial infections. These infections can become a major stumbling block to recovery and can exacerbate an already difficult situation. I strongly suggest that Type A and Type AB adopt a blood-building, immune system-enhancing protocol of additional vitamin supplementation a week or two prior to surgery. Vitamin B12, folic acid and supplemental iron should all be taken daily along with the already suggested levels of vitamins A and C. The concentration of vitamins needed here is difficult to squeeze out of the Type A and Type AB diets, so supplementation is best.

Floradix is a liquid source of iron and herbs that is both gentle on the digestive tract and highly assimilable. I highly recommend its use for iron supplementation since iron is usually an irritant to the digestive tracts of Type As and Type ABs. Floradix is found in most health food shops.

Avail yourselves of the two excellent immune-enhancing herbal teas, burdock root and echinacea. Begin to drink a few cups daily of these herbal teas at least a couple of weeks prior to surgery.

More than the other blood types, Type As and Type ABs often experience profound physical, mental and emotional stress because of the trauma of surgery. Relaxation techniques, such as meditation and visualization, can be of tremendous benefit to the more highly strung Type A and Type AB patient. By practising these techniques, you can have a profound influence upon your own healing process. Some anaesthesiologists will work with patients on visualizations while the patient is under anaesthesia. I urge you to ask your consultant about this. It's a perfect method for Type As.

AFTER THE SURGERY

Calendula succus (marigold) is used to help the wound heal and keep it clean. A solution of this homeopathic herb, a form of the marigold flower, is a wonderful healer for all cuts and scrapes in general. The juice has mild antibiotic properties and can be left on after application. Be sure you buy the juice (or *succus*) and not the *calendula* tincture, which has a high alcohol content. The tincture will really sting if you try to clean a wound with it.

As your incision heals and the stitches or staples are removed, a topical vitamin E preparation will minimize scar tissue formation and skin tightening. Many people just snip open a vitamin E capsule and smear it on, but oral supplements aren't formulated for use in skin healing. Use a topical cream or lotion blended specifically for this purpose.

LISTEN TO YOUR BLOOD TYPE

There are many vitamins and herbal supplements that aid the body in both defending and healing itself. The recommended surgical supplementation is just the minimum you should do to protect and strengthen yourself.

Each of the blood type diets contain pertinent information that allows you to make reasoned choices about what you should and should not allow yourself to eat and drink. All of these choices can have a profound effect on your health and the quality of your life.

By making knowledgeable choices about what is best for your body, you will be able to dramatically affect the course of both your treatment and recovery from surgery. This not only grants you greater control over your present circumstances, but enables you to ensure your future health.

Everyone can achieve benefits from an awareness of the blood type connection. It makes sense. It also solves the puzzle of why some people do very well with conventional treatments, while others suffer complications and pain. I urge you to make sure you are someone who does well.

9
Blood Type: A Power Over Disease

EVERYONE WHO GETS sick wants to know 'Why me?' Despite our enormous technological advances, we often have no certain answer to that question.

It has become clear, however, that there are individuals who are more prone to certain diseases because of their blood type. Perhaps this is the missing link – the way we can understand the cellular causes of disease, and devise more effective ways to combat and eliminate it.

Why Some People are Susceptible and Some are Not
Can you remember being young and having a close friend who wanted you to do something that you were reluctant to do? Take a puff of a forbidden cigarette? Sneak a drink of whisky from your father's drinks cabinet? Did you take that puff? Drink that whisky?

If you did, you demonstrated your susceptibility – your lack of resistance – to the suggestion of a friend.

Susceptibility, or lack of resistance, is the basic issue with most disease. Many microbes have the ability to mimic the antigens which are considered friendly by the security force of a particular blood type. These clever mimics bypass the security guards and gain entry. Once in the system, they quickly overwhelm it and take control.

Don't you ever wonder why one person stays perfectly healthy while everyone else is falling prey to the latest cold or flu? It is because the healthy person's blood type is not susceptible to those particular invaders.

The Blood Type Connection

There are many causal factors for disease that are clearly influenced by blood type. For instance, Type As with a family history of cardiovascular disease should examine their diets very carefully. Red meats and saturated fats of all kinds are poor choices for a digestive tract ill-suited to processing them, and which produces higher levels of both triglycerides and cholesterol in Type As. The friendly Type A immune system is also more prone to cancer, since it has a hard time recognizing foes.

Type Os, as I've said, are very sensitive to the agglutinating lectin found in whole wheat. This lectin interacts with the lining of the Type O intestinal tract and produces additional inflammation. If you're Type O and suffer from Crohn's disease, colitis, or irritable bowel syndrome, wheat acts like a poison in your system. Although the Type O immune system is generally hardy, it is also limited. Original Type Os had fewer microbes to conquer, and the blood type does not adapt easily to the complex viruses prevalent today.

The disease profiles of Type Bs are independent of Type O and Type A by virtue of the idiosyncratic B antigens. They tend to be susceptible to slow-moving, sometimes bizarre, viral diseases that don't manifest themselves for many years – like multiple sclerosis and rare neurological ailments – sometimes triggered by the lectins in foods such as chicken and corn.

Type ABs have the most complex disease profile, since they possess both A-like and B-like antigens. Most of their disease susceptibilities are A-like, so if you had to categorize them you would say they are more A than B.

The blood type connection between good health and disease is a potent tool in our search for the best way to treat the body as it is *meant* to be treated.

Still, I must add a caveat, for fear you think that I am proposing a magic formula. There are many factors in every individual life that contribute to disease. It would be overly simplistic and certainly foolish to suggest that blood type is the sole determining factor. If a Type O, a Type A, a Tybe B and a Tybe AB each drank a cup of arsenic, each of them would die. By the same token, if four people of different blood types were all heavy smokers, they would all be susceptible to lung cancer.

The blood type information is not a panacea, but a meaningful refinement that will enable you to function at your peak.

* * *

Let's turn to the most common and troubling diseases and conditions for which we can identify a blood type relationship. Some blood type-disease relationships are more clearly defined than others. We are still learning. But every day blood type is revealed as a dominating factor – the previously missing link in our quest for health.

Categories

- Ageing diseases
- Allergies
- Autoimmune disorders
- Blood disorders
- Cardiovascular disease
- Childhood illnesses
- Diabetes
- Digestive illnesses
- Infections
- Liver disease
- Skin disorders
- Women/reproduction

(Note: Cancer is such a complex topic that I have devoted an entire chapter to it, beginning on p. 295)

AGEING DISEASES

All people age, no matter what their blood type. But why do we age – and can we slow down the process? These questions have fascinated humans for as long as we can remember. The promise of a Fountain of Eternal Youth has appeared in every century. Today, with our sophisticated medical technology and our increased knowledge of the factors that contribute to ageing, we are closer to an answer.

But there's another question: why do individual ageing patterns differ so greatly? Why does the 50-year-old runner, lean and seemingly fit, drop dead of a heart attack, while the 89-year-old woman, who has never broken into a sweat in her life, remains hale and hearty? Why do some people develop Alzheimer's disease, or dementia, while others do not? At what age does physical deterioration become inevitable?

We understand some pieces of the puzzle. Genetics play a role; unique variations in chromosomes contribute to susceptibilities that cause deterioriation more rapidly in one person than in another. But these studies are incomplete.

I have discovered, however, a critical link between blood type and ageing – specifically, a correlation between the agglutinating action of lectins and the two biggest physiological associations of ageing – kidney failure and brain deterioration.

As we age we experience a gradual drop in kidney function so that by the time the average person reaches 72, his or her kidneys are operating at only 25 per cent of their capacity. Your kidney function is a reflection of the volume of blood that gets cleaned and recirculated into your bloodstream. This filtering system is very delicate – large enough for the various fluid elements of blood to go through, but small enough to prevent whole cells from passing through.

Consider the way the agglutinating actions of lectins gum up the works. Because the kidneys play a central role in the filtration of blood, the actions of many lectins can, over time, upset the delicate process. Those lectins that find their way into the bloodstream end up agglutinating and lodging in the kidneys. The process is similar to having a clogging drain. Over time, the filtration system ceases to function. As more and more agglutination occurs, less and less blood is able to be cleaned. It is a slow process, but ultimately deadly. Kidney failure is one of the leading causes of physical deterioration in the elderly.

The second large physiological association of ageing occurs in the brain. Here lectins play an equally destructive role. Scientists have observed that the difference between an old brain and a young brain is that in an old brain many elements of neurones get tangled up. This tangling, which leads to dementia and overall deterioration (and might even be a factor in Alzheimer's disease), occurs very gradually over the decades of adult life.

How do lectins reach the brain? Remember, lectins come in all shapes and sizes; some are small enough to pass the blood–brain barrier. Once they reach the brain they begin to agglutinate the blood cells, gradually interfering with neurone activity. The process occurs over many decades, but eventually the neurones get tangled enough to have an effect on brain function.

It is clear to me that by reducing or eliminating the most harmful lectins from your diet, you can maintain healthier kidneys and brain function for a longer period of time. That is why some very old people remain mentally sharp and physically active.

A third way that lectins contribute to ageing is their effect on our hormonal functions. It is well documented that as people age they have greater trouble absorbing and metabolizing nutrients. That's one reason why elderly people often become malnourished, even when they are eating their normal diets. Dietary guidelines normally call for added supplementation for the elderly. But if agglutinating lectins are not overwhelming the system and interfering with hormonal activity, it is likely that elderly people can absorb nutrients just as effectively as when they were younger.

I am not proposing that the blood type connection is a formula for reversing the effects of ageing that have already occurred. But you can reduce cellular damage by reducing your lectin intake at *any* age. Most of all, your Blood Type Plan is designed to slow down the process of ageing during your entire adult life.

ALLERGIES

Food Allergies
In my opinion, no area of alternative medicine is as shot full of humbug as the concept of food allergy. Complex and expensive tests are conducted on practically every patient, resulting in a list of foods to which that person is 'allergic'.

My own patients habitually term any reaction to something

they've eaten a 'food allergy', although most of the time it is not an allergy they are describing, but rather a food intolerance. If you have a problem with lactose in milk, for example, you are not allergic to it; you lack an enzyme to break it down. You are lactose intolerant, not lactose allergic. This intolerance does not necessarily mean you'll get sick if you drink milk. Type Bs who are lactose intolerant, for example, are often able to gradually introduce milk products into their diets. There are also products that add the lactose enzyme to milk products, making them more palatable for the intolerant.

A food allergy is a very different type of reaction that occurs, not in the digestive tract, but in the immune system. Your immune system literally creates an antibody to a food. The reaction is swift and severe – rashes, swelling, cramps or other specific symptoms that indicate your body is struggling to rid itself of the poisonous food.

Not everything in nature is perfectly cut and dried. Occasionally I'll come across a person who is allergic to a food that is on his blood type diet. The solution: simply remove the offending food. The main point is that you have more to fear from the hidden lectins entering your system than you do from food allergies. You may not feel sick when you eat the food, but it is nonetheless affecting your system. Type As should also be aware that if they produce excessive mucus, it may appear to be an allergy when they should actually be avoiding mucus-producing foods.

Asthma and Hay Fever

Type Os win the allergy sweepstakes hands down! They are more likely to be asthma sufferers, and even hay fever, the bane of so many lives, appears to be specific to Type O blood. A wide range of pollens contain lectins which stimulate the release of the powerful histamines, and then boom! – itching, sneezing, runny nose, wheezing, coughing, red, watery eyes – all the allergy symptoms.

Many food lectins, especially wheat, interact with immunoglobin-E (IgE) antibodies found in the blood. These antibodies stimulate white blood cells called basophiles to release not only histamines, but other powerful chemical allergens called kinins. These can cause severe allergic reactions such as the swelling of throat tissues and constricting of the lungs.

Asthma and hay fever sufferers do best when they follow the diet recommended for their blood type. For example, Type Os who eliminate wheat often relieve many of their symptomatic behaviours, such as sneezing, respiratory problems, snoring or persistent digestive disorders.

Type As have a different problem. Instead of environmental reactions, they often develop stress-related asthma as a result of their intense stress profiles (see the Type A Plan). When Type As suffer from excessive production of mucus caused by poor dietary choices, it makes the stress-related asthma worse. Type As, as you will remember, naturally produce copious amounts of mucus, and when they eat foods that are mucus-producing (like dairy products), they suffer from over-production of mucus which exacerbates respiratory problems. In this case, when Type As are careful to avoid the problematic foods, and when the causes of the stress are addressed positively, their asthmatic condition always improves or is eliminated.

By design, Type Bs are not prone to developing allergies. They have a high allergy threshold, unless they eat the wrong foods. For example, the Type B-poisoning chicken and corn lectins will trigger allergies in even the most resistant of this blood group.

Type ABs seem to have the least problem with allergies, probably because their immune systems are the most environmentally friendly. The combination of A-like and B-like antigens give Type ABs a double dose of antigens with which to fight environmental intrusion.

AUTOIMMUNE DISORDERS

Autoimmune disorders are immune system breakdowns. Immune defences develop what amounts to severe amnesia; they no longer recognize themselves. The result is that they run amok, making auto-antibodies that attack their own tissues. These warlike auto-antibodies think they are protecting their turf, but in reality they are destroying their own organs and inciting inflammatory responses. Examples of autoimmune disease include rheumatoid arthritis, lupus nephritis, ME (Chronic Fatigue Syndrome/ Epstein-Barr), multiple sclerosis, and amyotrophic lateral sclerosis (ALS/Lou Gehrig's Disease).

Arthritis

Type Os are the predominant sufferers of arthritis, an autoimmune disorder. Type O immune systems are environmentally intolerant, and there are many foods – grains and potatoes among them – whose lectins produce inflammatory reactions in their joints.

My father observed many years ago that Type Os tended to develop a 'gritty' sort of arthritis, a chronic deterioration of the bone cartilage. This is the kind of arthritic condition called osteoarthritis, typically found in the elderly. Type As tend to develop a 'puffy' arthritis, which it the more acute rheumatoid form of the disease – a painful and debilitating breakdown of multiple joints.

In my own experience, most people who suffer from rheumatoid arthritis are Type As. The anomaly of Type As, with their immunologically tolerant systems, the development of this form of arthritis may be related to A-specific lectins. Laboratory animals injected with A-specific lectins developed inflammation and joint destruction that was indistinguishable from rheumatoid arthritis.

There is also the probable stress connection. Some studies show that people with rheumatoid arthritis tend to be more highly strung and less emotionally resilient. When they have poor coping-mechanisms for life stress the disease progresses more rapidly. This makes sense in view of what we know about the stress factor, and about Type As who are inherently highly strung. Type As with rheumatoid arthritis should certainly incorporate daily relaxation techniques, as well as calming exercises.

ME (Chronic Fatigue Syndrome)

In recent years, I have treated many people who suffered from the baffling disease called ME or Chronic Fatigue Syndrome.

The primary symptom is great tiredness. Other more advanced symptoms include painful muscles and joints, persistent sore throats, digestive problems, allergies and chemical sensitivities.

The most important thing I've learned from my research and clinical work is that ME may not be an autoimmune disease at all, but rather a liver disease. (I place it in this section because that's where people are accustomed to looking for it.)

Although ME masquerades as a virus or autoimmune disease, the root cause is more likely a problem of poor metabolism in the liver. In other words, the liver is unable to detoxify chemicals. To my reasoning, only this sort of liver problem could produce immunologic effects as well as effects characteristic of other systems, such as digestive or musculo-skeletal.

I've found that Type O ME patients, in particular, do very well on liquorice and potassium supplements, in addition to the Type O diet. Liquorice has many effects in the body, but in the liver it really shines. The bile ducts (where detoxification occurs) become more efficient, with greater protection against chemical damage. This preliminary removal of stress to the liver seems to positively influence the adrenals and blood sugar, increasing energy and a feeling of well-being. The blood type-specific exercise activities seem to also serve as a valuable guide to help return to appropriate forms of physical activity. (Note: do not use liquorice other than under a GP's supervision.)

* * *

Case History: ME
(*from Dr John Prentice, Everett, Washington, USA*)
Karen, 44: Type B

My colleague, Dr John Prentice, tried the Blood Type Plan for the first time on a patient with severe ME (Chronic Fatigue Syndrome). He wasn't totally convinced it would work, but all efforts to help his very sick patient had failed, and he contacted me when he heard of the work I was doing with ME patients.

Karen was a tough case. She had suffered terrible fatigue for her entire adult life, and had needed 12 hours of sleep every night since she was a teenager. She would steal naps when she could. For the last seven years her exhaustion prevented her from holding a job. In addition, her neck, shoulders and back were constantly in pain, and she suffered debilitating headaches. Recently, Karen had started experiencing terrible anxiety attacks, with heart palpitations so severe she would call for an ambulance. She felt her circulation, or even her whole body, was shutting down.

Karen was a wealthy woman, but most of her inheritance was spent on making the rounds of doctors. She had been to more than 50 doctors, both conventional and alternative, before she came to Dr Prentice.

Dr Prentice started Karen on a programme of strict adherence to the Type B diet, supplements and exercise regimen. Both he and Karen were astonished to see that within only a week she had a tremendous increase in energy. Within a few weeks, most of her symptoms were resolved.

Dr Prentice tells me that today Karen is a new person. 'It's like clockwork,' he says. 'When she eats "off" her diet, her body reminds her with severe symptoms, so she sticks with it closely.' He shared a letter she had written him: 'I have a whole new life. All my symptoms are practically gone and I hold two jobs, having great energy 14 hours a day consistently. I believe the diet is key to this tremendous change. I am extremely active and feel like nothing can stop me. Thank you so very much!'

* * *

Multiple Sclerosis and ALS (Lou Gehrig's Disease)

Both Multiple Sclerosis and ALS (amyotrophic lateral sclerosis) occur in blood Type B with very high frequency. It's an example of the Type B's tendency to contract unusual slow-growing viral and neurological disorders. The Type B association may explain why Jews, a high number of which are Type B blood, suffer these diseases more than others. Some researchers believe that Multiple Sclerosis and ALS are caused by a virus, contracted in youth, that has a B-like appearance. The virus cannot be combated by the Type B immune system since it is unable to produce anti-B antibodies. The virus grows slowly and without symptoms for twenty or more years after entering the system.

Type ABs are also at risk from these B-like diseases, since their bodies do not produce anti-B antibodies. Type O and Type A seem to be relatively immune by virtue of their strong anti-B antibodies.

* * *

Case history: Autoimmune disorder
Joan, 55: Type O

Joan, a middle-aged dentist's wife, was a classic example of the ravages of autoimmune disorders. She suffered from severe symptoms of chronic fatigue/EBV, arthritis, and tremendous discomfort caused by gas and bloating. Joan's digestive system was so disrupted that practically everything she ate caused bouts of diarrhoea. By the time she arrived in my office, she had been struggling with these conditions for more than a year. Needless to say, she was terrible weakened and in great pain. She was also very discouraged. Since autoimmune disorders can be difficult to pin down, many people (even some doctors) don't believe chronic fatigue sufferers are really sick. Imagine the humiliation and frustration of feeling deathly ill but having people tell you it's all in your head!

Worse still, Joan's doctors had experimented with a number of drug therapies, including steroids, which made her even sicker and contributed to her bloating. She had also been told to adopt a diet high in grains and vegetables, and to limit or eliminate red meat – exactly the opposite of what this Type O should have been doing.

Even though Joan's symptoms were severe, the treatment was fairly simple – a detoxification programme, the Type O Diet and a regimen of nutritional supplements. Within two weeks, Joan experienced significant improvement. By the six-month mark, she was feeling 'normal' again. To this day, Joan's energy level is good, her digestion is healthy and her arthritis only flares up when she indulges in the rare sandwich or ice-cream.

Case History: Lupus
(*from Dr Thomas Kruzel, ND, Gresham, Oregon, USA*)
Marcia, 30: Type A

My colleague, Dr Kruzel, was interested in trying the blood type treatments, but he was initially sceptical. It was a case of lupus nephritis which showed him the true value of serotyping (blood testing) for the treatment of disease.

Marcia, a frail young woman suffering from lupus, was carried into Dr Kruzel's office by her brother, after being discharged from the hospital intensive care unit. She had suffered kidney failure from circulating complexes related to her disease. Marcia had been on shunt dialysis for several weeks and was scheduled for renal transplantation within the next six months.

Dr Kruzel took her medical notes and learned that Marcia's diet was very high in dairy, wheat and red meat – all dangerous foods for a Type A person in her condition. He placed her on a strict vegetarian diet along with hydrotherapy and homeopathic preparations. Within two weeks, Marcia's condition had improved and her need for dialysis had decreased. Remarkably, within a two-month period, Marcia was taken completely off dialysis and her previously scheduled kidney transplant was cancelled. Three years later, she is still doing well.

* * *

BLOOD DISORDERS
It should come as no surprise that blood-related illnesses, like anaemia and clotting disorders, are blood type specific.

Pernicious Anaemia
Type As constitute the greatest number of pernicious anaemia sufferers, but the condition has nothing to do with the vegetarian Type A diet. Pernicious anaemia is the result of vitamin B12 deficiency, and Type As have the most difficulty absorbing B12 from the foods they eat. Type ABs also have a tendency towards pernicious anaemia, although not as great as Type As.

The reason for the deficiency is that the body's use of B12

requires high levels of stomach acid and the presence of intrinsic factor, a chemical produced by the lining of the stomach and responsible for B12's assimilation. Type As and Type ABs have lower levels of intrinsic factor than the other blood types, and they don't produce very much stomach acid. For this reason, most Type As and Type ABs who suffer from pernicious anaemia respond best when vitamin B12 is administered by injection. By eliminating the need for the digestive process to assimilate this vital and potent nutrient, it is made available to the body in a more highly concentrated way. This is a case where dietary solutions *alone* don't work, although Type As and Type ABs are able to absorb Floradix, a liquid iron and herb supplement.

Type Os and Type Bs tend not to suffer from anaemia; they have high stomach-acid levels and sufficient levels of intrinsic factor.

* * *

Case History: Anaemia
(*from Dr Jonathan V. Wright, MD, Kent, Washington, USA*)
Carol, 35: Type O

The blood type diets have begun to make their way into conventional medicine as I have shared them with my colleagues. Dr Wright was one who successfully used the diet to treat a woman with chronically low levels of iron in her blood. Carol had tried every available form of iron supplement with no success. Dr Wright tried a number of other treatments without success. The only thing that worked at all was injectable iron, but it was only a temporary solution. Her iron levels would inevitably drop again.

I had spoken to Dr Wright on an earlier occasion about my work with lectins and blood types, and he called me for more details. He decided to try the Type O diet for Carol. After eliminating the incompatible lectins, which may have been damaging her red blood cells, and adhering to a high animal protein diet, the levels of iron in Carol's blood started to rise, and previously ineffective supplementation started to help. Dr

Wright and I agreed that it was the agglutination of the intestinal tract by the incompatible food lectins that prevented the iron from assimilating.

* * *

Clotting Disorders

Type Os face the biggest problems when it comes to blood clotting. Most often, Type Os lack sufficient quantities of the various blood-clotting factors. This can have severe consequences, especially during surgery, or in situations where there is blood loss. Type O women, for example, tend to lose significantly more blood after childbirth than women of other blood types.

Type Os with a history of bleeding disorders and strokes should emphasize foods containing chloroyphyll to help modify their clotting factors. Chlorophyll is found in almost all green vegetables, and is available as a supplement.

Type As and Type ABs don't suffer clotting disorders, but their thicker blood can work to their disadvantage in other ways. Thicker blood is more likely to deposit plaque in the arteries – one reason why Type A and Type AB are more prone to cardiovascular disease. Type A and Type AB women might have problems with heavy clotting during their menstrual periods if they don't keep their diets under control.

Type Bs tend not to suffer from clotting disorders or thick blood. As long as they follow the Type B diet, their balanced systems work efficiently.

CARDIOVASCULAR DISEASE

Cardiovascular disease is epidemic in Western societies, with many factors to blame, including diet, lack of exercise, smoking and stress.

Is there a connection between your blood type and your susceptibility to cardiovascular disease?

When in the late 1960s the Framingham (Massachusetts) Heart Study examined the connection between blood type and heart disease, it found no clear-cut blood type distinction as to who gets heart disease. It did, however, discover a strong connection between blood type and who survives heart disease. The study found that Type O heart patients, between the ages of 39 and 72, had a much higher rate of survival than Type A heart patients in the same age group. This was especially true for men between the ages of 50 and 59.

Although the Framingham Heart Study did not explore this subject in depth, it does appear that the same factors involved in surviving heart disease also offer some protection against getting it in the first place. Given these factors, clearly there is a greater risk for Type As and Type ABs. Let's examine them.

The most significant factor is cholesterol, the primary causal factor in coronary artery disease. Most of the cholesterol in our bodies is produced in our livers, but there is an enzyme called phosphatase manufactured in the small intestine that is responsible for the absorption of dietary fats. High-alkaline phosphatase levels, which speed the absorption and metabolism of fats, lead to low cholesterol levels in the blood. Type O blood normally has the highest matural levels of this enzyme. In Type B, Type AB, and Type A, the alkaline phosphatase enzyme is seen in ever declining levels, with Type B having the highest level after Type O.

Another element to Type Os' high survival rate is blood-clotting factors. As we discussed earlier, Type Os have fewer clotting factors in their blood. This defect in Type O blood may actually work to their advantage, as this essentially thinner blood is less likely to deposit the plaque that will clog the arterial flow. On the other hand, Type As, and to a slightly lesser extent, Type ABs, have a consistently higher level of serum cholesterol and triglycerides than do Type O and Type B blood.

* * *

Case history: Heart disease
Wilma, 52: Type O

Wilma was a 52-year-old Lebanese woman with advanced cardiovascular disease. When I first examined her, she had recently come out of the hospital after receiving a balloon angioplasty, a procedure used to treat clogged coronary arteries. She told me that her cholesterol had been over 350 at the time of the original diagnosis (normal is 200–220), and three of her arteries had blockages of over 80 per cent.

Since Wilma was Type O, her illness was a bit of a surprise, considering that Type Os normally have a lower-than-average incidence of heart disease. She was also quite a bit younger than most women with such severe blockages; women tend not to develop heart disease until long after the menopause.

Wilma had always eaten the traditional Lebanese diet, including lots of olive oil, fish and grains, which most doctors feel is beneficial to the circulatory system. However, five years earlier, at the age of 47, she began to experience pain in her neck and arms. Heart disease didn't even occur to her! She assumed the pain was arthritis, and was stunned when her doctor diagnosed her problem as angina pectoris, pain caused from an inadequate blood and oxygen supply to the heart muscle.

After her angioplasty, Wilma's cardiologist advised her to begin taking a cholesterol-lowering drug. A well-read health consumer, Wilma worried about long-term problems with drug therapy, and she wanted to try a natural approach before opting for the drug. That's when she came to me.

Since Wilma was Type O, I suggested that she add lean red meat to her diet. In light of her condition, she was understandably nervous about eating foods which are usually restricted in people with high cholesterol or heart disease. She immediately consulted her cardiologist who was – no surprise – appalled at the idea. Again, he urged her to take the drug. But Wilma was serious about avoiding drug therapy, so she decided to follow the Type O diet for three months, and then have a cholesterol check.

Wilma confirmed many of my theories about susceptibility to high cholesterol. Through heredity or by other mechanisms, people often have high levels of cholesterol in their blood in spite of a severely restricted diet. Usually they have some defect in the manipulation of the internal cholesterol metabolism. My suspicion is that when Type Os eat a lot of certain carbohydrates (usually wheat products) it modifies the effectiveness of their insulin, resulting in it becoming more potent and longer lasting.

From the increased insulin activity, the body stores more fat in the tissues and elevates the triglyceride (blood fat) stores.

In addition to advising Wilma to increase the percentage of red meats in her diet, I also helped her find substitutes for the large amounts of wheat she was consuming, and prescribed an extract of hawthorn (a herb used as a tonic for the heart and arteries) and a low dose of niacin, a B vitamin, which helps reduce cholesterol levels.

Wilma was an executive secretary with a stressful job and she did very little exercise. She was intrigued when I described the relationship between stress and physical activity in people with Type O blood, as well as the relationship between stress and heart disease. She had never been a regular exerciser, so hardly knew where to begin. I started her on a walking programme to gradually increase her aerobic fitness. After a couple of weeks, Wilma reported that walking was a godsend; she'd never felt better.

Within six months Wilma's cholesterol plummeted, without medication, to 187, where it stabilized. She was elated to have cholesterol in the normal range. It had seemed impossible. The naturopath intern working in my office was astounded and perplexed. All conventional evidence indicates that people with high cholesterol should avoid red meats, yet Wilma flourished. Blood type was the missing link.

Case history: Dangerously high cholesterol
John, 23: Type O

John, a recent college graduate, had a rocketing cholesterol level, high triglycerides and high blood sugar. These were very unusual symptoms in a young man, especially since he was Type O. As there was a strong history of heart disease, his parents were naturally alarmed. After extensive check-ups by consulting cardiologists, John was told that his genetic predisposition was so overwhelming that even cholesterol-reducing medication would be useless. In effect, John was told that he was destined to develop coronary artery disease – sooner, rather than later.

In the office, John seemed depressed and lethargic. He

complained of severe fatigue. 'I used to love to work out,' he said, 'but now I just don't have the energy.' John also suffered from frequent sore throats and swollen glands. His past history revealed mononucleosis and two separate incidences of Lyme disease (a tick-borne infection endemic in the eastern US).

John had been following a vegetarian diet which had been for some time prescribed by his cardiologist. He admitted, however, that he was feeling worse on this diet, not better.

After only a few weeks on the Type O diet, however, the results were amazing. Within five months, John's serum cholesterol, triglycerides and blood sugar all dropped to normal levels. A repeat blood profile after three months revealed similar results.

If John continued to follow the Type O diet, exercise regularly and take nutritional supplements there was a good chance that he would beat the odds of his genetic inheritance.

* * *

High Blood Pressure

Constantly at work within us is the dynamic force of our beating hearts, rhythmically pumping through our bodies. The process is normally so smooth that we rarely think much about it. That's why high blood pressure (or hypertension) is called the silent killer. It's possible to have dangerously high blood pressure and be entirely unaware of it.

When blood pressure is taken, two numbers are read. The systolic reading (the number on top) measures the pressure within the arteries as your heart beats out blood. The diastolic reading (the number on the bottom) measures the pressure present within the arteries as your heart rests between beats. Normal systolic pressure is 120, and normal diastolic pressure is 80 – or an overall reading of 120 over 80 (120/80). High blood pressure (or hypertension) is 140/90 under age 40, and 160/95 over age 40.

Depending on the severity and duration, untreated high blood pressure opens the door to a host of problems, including heart attacks and strokes.

Little is known about the blood type-related risk factors for hypertension. However, hypertension often occurs in conjunction with heart disease, so Type As and Type ABs should be particularly vigilant.

Hypertension carries the same risk factors as cardiovascular disease. Smokers, diabetics, post-menopausal women, the obese, the sedentary and people in stressful positions, should pay extra attention to the details of their blood type programme – especially to the diet and exercise recommendations.

* * *

Case History: Hypertension
Bill, 54: Type A

Bill was a middle-aged bond trader with high blood pressure. When I first saw him in my office in March 1991, his blood pressure was an almost explosive 150/105 to 135/95. It didn't take long to find clues to these numbers in his incredibly stressful life, which included a partnership in a high-powered firm and a host of domestic problems. Against his doctor's urging, Bill had discontinued his blood pressure medication because it made him dizzy and constipated. He wanted to try a more natural therapy, but it had to be done immediately.

I placed Bill on a Type A diet – a huge adjustment for this burly Italian. And I immediately began to address Bill's stress with the exercise regimen designed for Type As. He was initially embarrassed about doing yoga and relaxation exercises, but was soon converted when he realized how much calmer and more positive he felt.

At his first visit, Bill also confided that he had a special problem of a different nature. He and his partners were in the process of negotiating their office health plan, and if his hypertension was detected at his insurance physical, his firm would have to pay a much higher premium. Using the stress reduction techniques, the Type A diet and several botanicals, Bill was able to sail through his insurance physical.

* * *

CHILDHOOD ILLNESSES

A large number of the patients who come through my office are children suffering from a host of ailments – from chronic diarrhoea to repeated ear infections. Their mothers are usually on the verge of becoming frantic. Some of my most satisfying results have come with children.

Conjunctivitis

Conjunctivitis, commonly called 'pink eye', is usually caused by the transmission of the *staphylococcus* bacteria from one child to another. Type A and Type AB children are more susceptible to conjunctivitis than are Type O or Type B, probably because of their naturally weaker immune systems.

Antibiotic creams or eye drops are conventionally used to treat the condition, but a soothing and surprising alternative is a freshly-cut slice of tomato. (Don't try this with tomato juice!) The freshly-cut tomato water contains a lectin which can agglutinate and destroy the *staphylococcus* bacteria. The slight acidity of the tomato appears to closely resemble the acidity of the eye's own secretions. Squeezing the watery juice of a fresh tomato on a gauze pad and applying it to the affected eye is also very soothing.

This is one example of how the same lectins in a food that make it dangerous to eat, can be highly beneficial to treat an illness. Later, we'll discuss other examples of the ways in which lectins play a dual role in our systems – especially in the war against cancer.

Diarrhoea

Diarrhoea can be a disturbing and dangerous condition for children. Not only is it debilitating and terribly uncomfortable, but it can lead to severe dehydration, causing weakness and fever.

Most childhood diarrhoea is diet-related, and here the blood type diets offer very specific guidelines about which foods trigger digestive problems for each blood type.

Type O children often experience mild to moderate diarrhoea in reaction to eating dairy products.

Type A and Type AB children are prone to *Giardiasis lamblia*, more commonly known as Montezuma's Revenge, because the parasite mimics A qualities.

Type B children will contract diarrhoea if they overindulge in wheat products, or in reaction to eating chicken and corn.

If the diarrhoea is caused by food-related intolerance or allergy, a child will often exhibit other symptoms, ranging from dark, puffy circles under the eyes to eczema, psoriasis or asthma. Unless diarrhoea is the result of a more serious condition, such as a parasitic infection, partial intestinal blockage or inflammation, it usually corrects itself with time. If a child's stool contains blood or mucus, however, seek immediate medical attention. Acute diarrhoea might also be infectious; it is best to institute scrupulous standards of cleanliness to protect the rest of the family from contagion.

To restore a child's proper balance of fluids during bouts of diarrhoea, restrict fruit juice. Instead, feed the child vegetable or meat stocks in soups. Yogurt with active *L. acidophilus* cultures helps to maintain the good bacteria in the intestinal tract.

Ear Infections
Perhaps as many as four out of every ten children under the age of six have chronic ear infections. By chronic, I mean five, ten, fifteen, even twenty infections every winter season, one after the other. Most of these children have allergies to both environmental and food-based particles. The best solution is the blood type diet.

The conventional protocol for ear infections is antibiotic therapy. But it obviously fails when there is a chronic infection. If we attack the underlying causes of the problem first instead of trotting out the most currently fashionable nostrum – and by this I mean the ever more sophisticated and newest classes of antibiotics – we have an opportunity to allow the body to mount its own powerful response. For starters, it is helpful to know the blood type susceptibilities.

Children who are Type A and Type AB have greater problems with mucus secretions from improper diet – a factor in ear infections. In Type A children, dairy products are usually the culprit, whereas Type AB may experience sensitivities to sweetcorn in addition to milk. In general, these kids are also more likely to have throat and respiratory problems, which can often move into the ears. Because the immune systems of Type A and Type AB children are tolerant of a wider range of bacteria, some of their problems stem from the lack of an aggressive response to the infectious organism. Several studies have shown that ear fluids of children with a history of chronic ear infections lack specific chemicals called complement which are needed to attack and destroy the bacteria. Another study shows that a serum lectin called mannose binding protein is missing in the ear fluids of children with chronic infections. This lectin apparently binds to mannose sugars on the surface of the bacteria and agglutinates them, allowing for their faster removal. Both of these important immune factors eventually do develop in their proper amounts, which may help explain why the frequency of ear infections gradually lessens as the child ages.

In addition to diet, treating Type A and Type AB children with ear infections almost always involves enhancing their immunity. The simplest way to enhance the immunity of any child is to cut down on their intake of sugar. Numerous studies have shown that sugar depresses the immune system, making the body's white blood cells sluggish and disinclined to attack invading organisms.

Naturopaths have for many years made use of a mild herbal immune stimulant, echinacea (*Echinacea purpurea*). Originally used by Native Americans, echinacea has the extraordinary properties of being both safe and effective in boosting the body's immunity against bacteria and viruses. Since many of the immune functions which echinacea enhances are dependent on adequate levels of vitamin C, I often prescribe an extract of vitamin-C rich rose-hips. In the last three years I have been using an extract of Western larch tree as a sort of super-echinacea. This product was originally developed out of the paper-pulping industry and contains much more concentrated active components than echinacea. In my opinion, this product is an exciting new development which has revolutionized my treatment of a variety of immune deficiencies, including ear infections. I'm sure you'll be hearing much more about it in the very near future.

Ear infections are terribly painful for a child, and not too pleasant for the parents, either. Most of these infections are a buildup of noxious fluids and gases into the middle ear because of an obstructed connecting pipe, the Eustachian tube. This tube can become swollen because of allergic reactions, weakness in the tissues surrounding it or infections.

Many parents have grown frustrated by the increasing inability of antibiotics to work on ear infections. There is a reason why this happens. A baby's first ear infection is typically treated with a mild antibiotic such as Amoxicillin. With the child's next ear infection, Amoxicillin is given again. Eventually, the ever more resistant infection returns, and *Amoxicillin* is no longer effective. The escalation phenomenon – the process of using stronger and stronger drugs and ever more invasive treatments – has begun.

When antibiotics no longer work, and the painful infections continue, a myringotomy is performed. This is a process in which tiny tubes called grommets are surgically implanted through the eardrum to increase the drainage of fluid from the middle ear into the throat.

When I treat chronic ear infections, I focus on ways to prevent recurrences. It is useless to try and resolve one episode with a quick dose of antibiotics when you know another ear infection is warming up within. Almost always, I find a solution in the diet.

I see many children in my practice, representing all blood types. I've found that any child can contract chronic ear infections if he eats foods that react poorly in his system. I have never seen a case where there wasn't an obvious connection to a child's favourite food.

Type O and Type B children seem to develop ear infections less frequently, and when they do occur, they are usually easy to treat. More often than not, a change in diet is sufficient to eliminate the problem.

In Type B children, the culprit is usually a viral infection which then leads to infection with a bacteria called *hemophilus*, to which Type Bs are usually susceptible. The dietary remedy involves restricting tomatoes, sweetcorn and chicken. The lectins in these foods react with the surface of the digestive tract, causing swelling and mucus secretion, which usually carries over to the ears and throat.

My personal feeling is that ear infections can be prevented in Type O children simply by breast-feeding instead of bottle feeding. Breast-feeding for at least a year allows a child's immune system and digestive tract time to develop. Type O children will also avoid ear infections if they are taken off wheat and dairy products. They're unusually sensitive to these foods at an early age, but their immunity is easily augmented by the use of high-value proteins such as fish and lean red meats.

Dietary changes are often difficult in households with children who suffer repeated ear infections. Their misery often tempts the anxious parent to let them eat whatever they wish, thinking that it will comfort the child. Many of these kids wind up being picky eaters, eating only a very narrow range of foods, and often the very foods that are provoking the child's illness!

* * *

Case history: Ear infection
Tony, 7: Type B

Tony was a seven-year-old boy who suffered from repeated ear infections. When his mother first brought him to my office in January 1993, she was frantic. Tony would develop a new ear infection immediately after he stopped the antibiotic used to treat his previous infection – at the rate of 10–15 per winter season. He had had grommet treatment twice, but to no avail. This was a perfect example of a child on the antibiotic treadmill – escalating levels of antibiotics with fewer results.

My initial questions to Tony's mother were about his diet. She was a bit defensive. 'Oh, I don't think that's the problem,' she told me, 'we eat very well – lots of chicken and fish, fruits and vegetables.' Tony told me his favourite foods were chicken nuggets and corn-on-the-cob. I realized that the problem was that he was allergic to chicken and sweetcorn as he was a Type B. I explained the blood type connection and, although Tony's mother was unconvinced, I suggested she feed Tony the Type B diet for two or three months to see what would happen.

The rest, as they say, is history. Over the next two years Tony did very well, usually developing a single ear infection per season – as opposed to his previous rate of 10–15. These isolated infections were easy to treat either with naturopathic methods, or a gentle low-strength antibiotic.

* * *

Hyperactivity and Learning Disabilities
There are a variety of different causes for attention deficit disorders (ADD), and we still need much more information before we can make a conclusive blood type connection. We can, however, gain some insight from our knowledge of how different blood types respond to their environments. For example, my father has observed over 35 years of practice that Type O children are happier, healthier and more alert when they're given the opportunity to exercise to their maximum potential. A Type O child with ADD should be encouraged to exercise as much as possible. This might include additional gym classes, team sports or gymnastics. Type A and Type AB children, on the other hand, seem to benefit from activities which encourage the development of sensory and tactile skills, such as sculpting or artwork, and from basic relaxation techniques, such as deep breathing. Type B children do well with swimming and calisthenics.

There is some speculation among researchers that ADD is the result of sugar metabolism being out of sync, or allergies to dyes or other chemicals. There is no real conclusion that can be drawn at this point, although I've noticed that ADD children tend to be incredibly fussy eaters – which suggests a dietary connection.

I recently discovered an interesting connection that might more strongly tie Type O children to ADD. A Type O child was brought to me who suffered from both ADD and mild anaemia. I placed him on a high-protein diet and gave him supplements of vitamins B12 and folic acid, and the anaemia cleared up. But his mother also noticed a decided improvement in her child's attention span. I've subsequently treated several Type O ADD children with low doses of these vitamins and have seen improvements ranging from the slight to the dramatic.

If your child has ADD, talk to a nutrition professional about adding supplements of vitamin B12 and folic acid, in addition to the blood type diet.

Strep Throat, Mononucleosis and Mumps

Because the early symptoms of mononucleosis and the symptoms of strep throat are similar, it is often difficult for parents to differentiate between the two. A child with either illness may exhibit one or more of the following symptoms: sore throat, malaise, fever, chills, headache, swollen glands or swollen tonsils. A blood test and throat culture will be needed to determine which illness is causing the problem.

Strep throat, caused by the *streptococcal* organism, is a bacterial infection. It often has the additional symptoms of nasal discharge, cough, earaches, white or yellow patches on the back of the throat and a rash which starts on the neck and chest and spreads to the abdomen and extremities. Diagnosis of strep throat is based on clinical symptoms and a throat culture. The standard treatment includes antibiotics, bed rest and aspirin and fluids for aches and fever.

Once again, the focus is on treating the immediate infection, not on solving the larger and more long-term health issues. The standard therapy is ineffective, especially when your child suffers repeat infections.

In general, Type O and Type B children contract strep throat more often than Type A and Type AB because of their increased vulnerability to bacterial infections. However, Type O and Type B also recover more easily and completely. Once the strep organism gets into the bloodstream of Type A and Type AB, it settles in and doesn't want to leave. Thus, Type A and Type AB children will have repeated infections.

There are naturopathic therapies that can help prevent recurrences. I have found that using a mouth rinse made from the herbs sage and golden seal is very effective in keeping the throat and tonsils free from strep. Golden seal contains a component called berberine which has been well-documented for its anti-strep activity. The problem with golden seal is that it has a distinctly bitter, weedy taste which children don't exactly relish. It is sometimes easier to purchase an inexpensive atomizer or spray-pump bottle and just spray the back of your child's throat a couple of times a day. In addition to the blood type diets, I often use nutritional supplements for immune support, in the form of additional beta-carotene, vitamin C, zinc and echinacea to help develop the child's resistance.

With the viral infection mononucleosis, Type O seems to be more susceptible than Type A, Type B or Type AB. Antibiotics are ineffective in the treatment of mononucleosis because it is caused by a virus, not a bacteria. Bed rest while the fever lasts and frequent rest intervals during the one-to-three week recovery period are recommended. Aspirin and adequate fluid intake is encouraged to decrease fever.

Type B children seem to be more at risk for developing severe mumps, a viral infection of the salivary glands under the chin and ears. Like many B-prone illnesses, this one has a neurological connection. If your child is Type B and/or Rh− and has the mumps, be alert for signs of neurological damage, particularly manifested in hearing problems.

DIABETES
The blood type diets can be effective in the treatment of Type I (childhood) diabetes, and in both the treatment and prevention of Type II (adult) diabetes.

Blood Type A and Type B are more prone to Type I diabetes, caused by a lack of insulin, the hormone manufactured by the pancreas which is responsible for allowing glucose to enter the cells of the body. The cause of insulin deprivation is the destruction of the beta cells of the pancreas, which are the only cells capable of producing insulin.

Although there is currently no effective natural treatment alternative for injectable insulin replacement therapy in Type I diabetics, one important natural remedy to consider using is

Quercetin, an antioxidant derived from plants. Quercetin has been shown to help prevent many of the complications stemming from lifelong diabetes, such as cataracts, neuropathy and cardiovascular problems. Talk with a nutritionist who is skilled in the use of phytochemicals before using any natural medicine for diabetes; it may be necessary to re-adjust the insulin dosage.

Type II diabetics typically have high levels of insulin in their bloodstreams, but their tissues lack sensitivity to insulin. This condition develops over time and is usually the result of poor diet. Type II diabetes is often observed in Type Os who have eaten dairy, wheat and sweetcorn products for many years; and in Type As who eat a lot of meat and dairy foods. Type II diabetics are usually overweight and often have high cholesterol and elevated blood pressure – signs of a lifetime of poor food choices and lack of exercise. In this respect, any blood type can develop Type II diabetes.

The only real treatment for Type II diabetes is diet and exercise. The relevant blood type diet and exercise regimen will achieve results if you stick to the guidelines. A high-potency vitamin B complex can also help to counter insulin intolerance. Again, check with a GP and nutritionist before using any substance to treat diabetes.

DIGESTIVE ILLNESSES

Constipation

Constipation occurs when the stools are unusually hard or a person's bowel patterns have changed and become less frequent. Most chronic constipation is caused by poor bowel habits and irregular meals, with a diet low in fibre and water content. Some other causes are a habitual use of laxatives, a rushed and stressful daily schedule and travel that requires abrupt adjustments of eating and sleeping patterns. Lack of physical exercise, acute illness, painful rectal conditions and some medications may also cause constipation.

Every blood type is susceptible to constipation given the circumstances. Constipation is not so much a disease as a warning light that something is not right with a digestive system. Most of the clues will be in a person's diet. Are you eating enough foods on your diet that are high in fibre content? Are you drinking enough fluids – in particular, water and juices? Are you exercising regularly?

Many people simply take a laxative when they're constipated. But that doesn't solve the natural systemic causes of constipation. The long-term solution is in the diet. However, Type A, Type B and Type AB can supplement their diets with fibrous unprocessed bran. Type Os, in addition to eating plenty of the fibrous fruits and vegetables in their diets, can take a supplement of butyrate, a natural bulk-forming agent as a substitute for bran which is not advised for them.

Crohn's Disease and Colitis

Crohn's disease and colitis are both inflammatory diseases of the bowel; the former of the small intestine and the latter of the lower colon and rectum. They are depleting, enervating diseases which add the elements of uncertainty, pain, blood loss and suffering to the process of elimination. Many food lectins can cause digestive irritation by attaching to the mucous membranes of the digestive tract. As many of the food lectins are blood type specific, it is possible for each blood type to develop the same problem from different foods.

In Type As and Type ABs, Crohn's disease and colitis often involve a major stress component. Anyone with Type A or Type AB blood suffering from inflammatory bowel disease should pay careful attention to their stress patterns. (Refer to the discussion of stress in the relevant blood type plan.)

Type Os tend to develop the more ulcerative form of colitis that causes bleeding with elimination. This is probably due to the lack of adequate clotting factors in their blood. Type As, Type ABs and Type Bs tend to develop more of a mucous colitis, which is not as bloody. In either case, follow the diet for your blood type. You will be able to avoid many of the food lectins which can aggravate the condition, and you may find your symptoms easing.

* * *

Case History: Irritable Bowel Syndrome (IBS)
Virginia, 26: Type O

I first examined Virginia, a 26-year-old woman with chronic bowel trouble, three years ago, after she had received extensive treatment from a variety of conventional gastroenterologists. Her problems included chronic irritable bowel syndrome with painful constipation, alternating with an unpredictable, almost explosive diarrhoea which made it difficult for her to leave the house. She also suffered from fatigue and low-grade chronic anaemia. Her previous doctors conducted an enormous amount of testing (to the tune of $27,000!) and could only suggest anti-spasmodic drugs and a daily dose of fibre. Food allergy testing was inconclusive. Virginia was a vegetarian, who followed a strict macrobiotic diet, and I immediately detected the foods in her diet that were causing her suffering. The absence of meat in her diet was a primary factor. She was also unable to properly digest the grains and pasta she was eating as a main course.

Since Virginia was Type O, I suggested a high-protein diet, including lean red meats, fish and poultry, and fresh fruits and vegetables. As the digestive tract of Type O does not tolerate most grains very well, I suggested that she avoid whole wheat altogether and severely limit her consumption of other grains.

Initially, Virginia was resistant to the idea of making these dietary changes. She was a vegetarian and truly believed that her current diet was healthier. But I urged her to look again. 'How has this diet helped you, Virginia?' I asked. 'You seem to be pretty sick.'

Eventually, I convinced her to try it my way for a limited period of time. In eight weeks Virginia returned looking hale and hearty, with a ruddy complexion. She boasted that her bowel problems were 90 per cent better. Blood tests showed a complete resolution of her anaemia, and she said her energy levels were almost back to normal. A second follow-up visit one month later resulted in Virginia being discharged from my care, completely free of bowel problems.

Case history: Crohn's Disease
Yehuda, 50: Type O

I first saw Yehuda, a middle-aged Jewish man, in July, 1992, for active Crohn's Disease. By that point he had already had several bowel surgeries to remove sections which were obstructing his small intestine. I put Yehuda on a wheat-free diet, with an emphasis on lean meats and boiled vegetables. I also give him a high-powered extract of liquorice and the fatty acid butyrate.

Yehuda's compliance was exemplary, a testament to the concerns both he and the family had for his health. For example, his wife, the daughter of a baker, baked him a special wheat-free bread. Yehuda took his diet and supplements all very seriously, including the liquorice.

Yehuda consistently improved from the start. To this day he continues to be asymptomatic, although he must still be careful about using certain grains and dairy products, as they bother his digestion. He never required the additional surgery that his gastroenterologist had said was inevitable.

Case History: Crohn's Disease
Sarah, 35: Type B

Sarah was a 35-year-old woman of Eastern European ancestry. She first came to my office in June 1993, for treatment of Crohn's Disease. She had already had several surgeries to remove scarred tissue from the bowel, was anaemic and suffered from chronic diarrhoea.

I prescribed a basic Type B diet, instructing that Sarah remove chicken and other lectin-containing foods specific to Type B. I also used supplemental liquorice and fatty acids as part of her protocol.

Sarah was very co-operative. Within four months, most of her digestive symptoms, including the diarrhoea, were eliminated. As she wanted to have more children, Sarah recently had surgery to remove scar tissue from her bowel which had attached to her uterus. Her surgeon told her that there were no signs of active Crohn's Disease anywhere in her abdominal cavity.

* * *

Food Poisoning

Anyone can get food poisoning. But certain blood types are naturally more susceptible because of their tendency towards a weakened immune system. In particular, Type A and Type AB are more likely to fall prey to salmonella food poisoning, which is usually the result of leaving food uncovered and unrefrigerated for long periods of time. Furthermore, the bacteria will be more difficult for Type A and Type AB to get rid of once they've found a home in their systems.

Type Bs, who are generally more susceptible to inflammatory diseases, are more likely to be severely affected when they eat food that is contaminated with the *Shigella* organism, a bacteria found on plants that causes dysentery.

Gastritis

Many people confuse gastritis with ulcers, but it is exactly the opposite. Ulcers are produced by hyperacidity – more common in Type O and Type B. Gastritis is caused by very low stomach acid content – common for Type A and Type AB. Gastritis occurs when the stomach acid gets so low it no longer functions as a microbial barrier. Without adequate levels of acid, microbes will live in the stomach and cause serious inflammation.

The best course of action that Type A and Type AB can take is to stress the more acidic food choices in their blood type diets.

Stomach and Duodenal Ulcers

It has been known since the early 1950s that peptic ulcer of the stomach is more common in Blood Type O, with the highest occurrence in Type O non-secretors. Type Os also have a higher rate of bleeding and perforation, which was not shown to be different between secretors and non-secretors. One reason is that Type Os have higher stomach acid levels and an ulcer-producing enzyme called pepsinogen.

More recent research has uncovered another reason why Type Os are prone to ulcers. In December 1993, researchers at Washington University School of Medicine in St Louis reported in the *Journal of Science* that people with Type O blood are a favourite target for the bacteria now known to cause ulcers. This bacteria, *H. pylori*, was found to be able to attach itself to the Type O antigen lining the stomach, and then work its way into the lining. As we've seen, the Type O antigen is the fucose sugar. The researchers found an inhibitor in breast milk which apparently blocked the attachment of the bacteria to the stomach surface. No doubt this is one of the many fucose sugars found in human breast milk.

The common seaweed bladderwrack is an inhibitor of *H. pylori*. The content of fucose in bladderwrack is so great that it factors into its Latin name – *Fucus vesiculosis*. Any Type O who suffers from ulcers, or wants to prevent them, should use bladderwrack because it will make the ulcer-causing bacteria, *H. pylori*, slide off the stomach lining.

* * *

Case history: Chronic stomach ulcers
Peter, 34: Type O

I first met Peter in April 1992. He had suffered from stomach ulcers since he was a child, and had used every conventional ulcer medication available, with little result. I began by prescribing the basic high-protein Type O diet, stressing that he avoid the wholewheat products that had always been a major part of his diet. I also prescribed a supplement of bladderwrack, and a combination medicine of liquorice and bismuth.

Within six weeks Peter had made considerable progress. On a follow-up visit to his gastroenterologist, he had a colonoscopy and heard the encouraging news that 60 per cent of his stomach lining now appeared normal. A second examination in June 1993 showed complete resolution of Peter's stomach ulcers.

INFECTIONS
Many bacteria prefer specific blood types. In fact, one study showed that over 50 per cent of 282 bacteria carried antigens of one blood type or another.

It has been observed that viral infections in general seem to be more frequent in Type Os because they do not possess any antigens. These infections are less frequent and milder in Type A, Type B and Type AB.

Acquired Immune Deficiency Syndrome (AIDS)

I have treated many people who were HIV-positive or had full-blown AIDS, and I have yet to find a clear-cut connection between blood type and susceptibility to HIV. Having said that, let's look at how the information in this book can be used to help people hold their own against the virus.

While all the blood types appear to be equally susceptible to AIDS, given the exposure, there are variations in their susceptibility to the opportunistic infections (such as pneumonia and tuberculosis) that their weakened immune systems are prey to.

If you are HIV-positive or have AIDS, modify your diet to encompass the suggestions that are specific to your blood type. For example, if you are Type O, begin to increase the amount of animal proteins in your diet and develop a physical training programme. Following the blood type programme will help to fully mobilize and optimize your immune functions by stressing the highest value foods for your particular needs. Be careful to limit your fat intake, choosing lean cuts of meat, because bowel parasites, common in people with AIDS, interfere with fat digestion and lead to diarrhoea. Also, avoid foods such as wheat which contain lectins that could further compromise your immune system and bloodstream.

Since many of the opportunistic infections cause nausea, diarroea and mouth sores, AIDS is often a wasting disease. Type As will need to work a little harder to be sure that their calorie intake is high, since many Type A foods are calorifically low. Rigorously eliminate any foods, like meat or dairy, that can cause digestive problems. Your immune system is already naturally sensitive; don't give the lectins a chance to get in and weaken you further. Meanwhile, increase your portions of 'good' Type A foods, such as tofu and seafood.

Type Bs should avoid the obvious problem foods, like chicken, sweetcorn and buckwheat. But you should also eliminate nuts, which are hard to digest, and reduce the amount of wheat products in your diet. If you are lactose intolerant, avoid dairy foods; even if you're not, dairy can be a digestive irritant for immune-compromised Type Bs. This is a case where the disease is contra-indicative of the favoured food.

Type ABs should limit their intake of lectin-rich beans and pulses and eliminate nuts from their diets. Your primary protein source should be fish, and there is a wide variety available to Type ABs. Occasional servings of meat and dairy are OK, but watch the fat. And limit your wheat consumption.

In general, whatever your blood type, you want to avoid lectins that could damage the cells of your immune system and bloodstream. These cells cannot be as easily replaced as they can in a healthy body. This cell-sparing aspect of the blood type diets makes them invaluable to the person with AIDS who has anaemia or low T-helper cells.

The blood type diets help to preserve your precious immune cells from unnecessary damage. This can be a critical difference, especially as there are still no successful treatments for HIV infection.

* * *

Case History: AIDS
Arnold, 46: Type AB

Arnold was a middle-aged businessman with AIDS. He was married and believed he had been infected with HIV 12 years earlier. When I first saw him, Arnold's T-cell count, the barometer of the virus's destruction, was 6, with normal being 650 to 1700. He had a skin condition called molluscum which is often seen in the final stage of AIDS, and he was painfully thin from months of diarroea and nausea.

Arnold decided to come to a naturopath as a desperate, last-ditch effort to stay alive. I could see in his face that he didn't really believe this would work either, and I couldn't promise him dramatic results because I didn't really know what to expect.

My first goal was to prevent any lectins that were toxic to the Type AB immune system from entering his body. Along with that, it was urgent that I halt Arnold's wasting so he would be strong enough to fight the infection.

I began by tailoring the Type AB diet to the special needs raised by AIDS. This included: the elimination of all poultry except turkey, the introduction of low-fat organic meats, seafood several times a week, rice, lots of vegetables and fruit. I reduced most of the beans and pulses, and eliminated butter, cream, processed cheese, corn and buckwheat. In addition, I prescribed immune-boosting herbs, in tablet and tea form, including alfalfa, burdock root, echinacea, ginseng and ginger.

Within three months, Arnold's molluscum had cleared up and he was back in the gym. To this day he continues to be asymptomatic, even though his T-cells have not increased. He works and leads a fairly active life. The doctors at the infectious disease centre of his hospital are amazed. This is a man without an immune system!

Case History: AIDS
Susan, 27: Type O

After learning that her husband was HIV-positive, Susan was tested. She was frantic when she learned that she also had HIV. Lab tests revealed a very low T-cell count. Susan begged me to help her; she didn't want to die, and she was afraid to take AZT or any other drug specified for HIV.

We began with a Type O diet, along with nutritional supplements and regular exercise, and I instructed Susan to follow the programme closely. A few months later, Susan called to report that her T-cell count was in the 800s (normal is 500–1700). She has been symptom-free ever since.

Since there is at present no cure for HIV or AIDS, we can't gauge how long Susan will continue to do well. I believe that the more we discover about the mysteries of the immune system, the closer we'll come to making AIDS a disease to live with, rather than a disease to die from.

Bronchitis and pneumonia

In general, Type A and Type AB have more bronchial infections than Type O and Type B. This may result from improper diets which produce excessive mucus in their respiratory passages. This mucus facilitates the growth of blood-type mimicking bacteria, such as the A-like *Pneumococcus* bacteria in Type A and Type AB, and the B-like *Hemophilus* bacteria in Type B and Type AB. (Since Type AB has both A-like and B-like characteristics, the risk is double.)

The blood type diets seem to substantially reduce the incidence of bronchitis and pneumonia for all blood types. However, we are just beginning to discover some other blood type connections that are not so easily remedied. For example, it appears that Type A children born to Type A fathers and Type O mothers die more frequently of bronchopneumonia in early life. It is thought that some form of *senitization* occurs at birth between the Type A infant and the mother's anti-A antibodies which inhibits the infant's ability to fight the *Pneumococcus* bacteria. There is no solid data yet to confirm the reason this occurs, but information of this kind can spark research interest in a potential vaccine. We'll have to gather much more data before we can make a valid scientific conclusion.

Candidiasis (common yeast infection)

Although the candidiasis organism shows no preference for blood type, I have noticed that Type A and Type AB have a tougher time eradicating a severe yeast overgrowth once the organism finds a home in their tolerant systems. Candidiasis becomes like the unwanted guest who won't leave. Type A and Type AB also develop more yeast infections after antibiotic usage, which makes sense because antibiotics destroy their already weakened defence systems.

Type Os, on the other hand, develop more of an allergic-type hypersensitivity to the candidiasis organism, especially if they eat too many grains. This has been the basis of a theory called the yeast syndrome and a variety of candida diets. These diets stress high protein and the avoidance of grains, but they tend to be generalized across blood types, when it is only Type Os who appear to have this yeast sensitivity. If you're Type A or Type AB, yeast avoidance won't do anything to prevent yeast infections, and you'll only further compromise your immune system.

In general, Type Bs are less prone to this organism, as long as they follow the Type B diet. If you are a Type B who has a history of candidiasis, cut down on your wheat consumption.

Cholera

A report from Peru recently published in the *Lancet* attributed the severity of a recent epidemic of cholera – an infection characterized by extreme diarrhoea with severe fluid and mineral depletion – to the high incidence of Type Os in the Peruvian population. Historically, the susceptibility of Type Os to cholera probably decimated the population of many of the ancient cities, leaving as survivors the more cholera-resistant Type As.

Common cold and flu

There are hundreds of different strains of cold virus, and it would be impossible to see blood type specificity in all of them. However, studies of British military recruits showed a slightly lower overall incidence of cold viruses in recruits who were Type A, which is consistent with our findings that Blood Type A was developed to be resistant to these common viruses.

Viruses also have less impact on Type AB. The A antigen, carried by both Type A and Type AB, blocks the attachment of various strains of flu to the membranes of the throat and respiratory passages.

Influenza, a more serious virus, also strikes Type O and Type B in preference to Type A and Type AB. In its early stages, influenza may share many of the symptoms of a common cold. However, the flu causes dehydration, muscle pains, and serious weakness.

The symptoms of a common cold or flu are miserable, but they are actually a sign that your immune system is trying to fight off the offending virus. While your immune system is doing its job, there are measures you can take that will make co-existence on the battlefield more comfortable:

1. Maintain general good health with adequate rest and exercise, along with learning to cope with the stresses of life. Stress is a major factor in the depletion of immune system resources. This may protect you from frequent infections and may even shorten the duration of the colds and flus you do get.

2. Follow the basic dietary protocol for your blood type. It will optimize your immune response and help shorten the course of your cold or flu.

3. Take extra vitamin C (250–500 mg), or increase the sources of vitamin C in your diet. Many people feel that taking small doses of the herb echinacea helps prevent colds, or at least helps to shorten their duration.

4. Increase the humidity in your room with a vaporizer or humidifier to prevent dryness in the throat and nasal tissue.

5. If your throat is sore, gargle with salt water. Half a teaspoon of ordinary table salt and a tall glass of warm water provides a soothing and cleansing rinse. Another good gargle, especially if you are prone to tonsillitis, is a tea of equal parts golden seal root (*Hydrastis canadensis*) and sage. Gargle with this mixture every few hours.

6. If your nose is runny or stuffy, use an antihistamine to reduce the reaction of tissues to the infecting virus and relieve nasal congestion. Be especially careful with antihistamines containing ephedrine, such as those found in health food shops and in some OTC decongestants. These can raise the blood pressure, keep you awake at night, and complicate prostate problems in men.

7. Antibiotics are not effective against viruses. If someone offers

you their leftover antibiotics, or if you have some around the house, don't take them.

Plague, typhoid, smallpox and malaria

Known from the Middle Ages as The Black Death, plague is a bacterial infection largely carried by rodents. Blood Type O people are more susceptible to plague. Although plague is rare in industrialized societies, it continues to be a problem in Third World countries. A recent report by the World Health Organization warned that we may be facing a crisis in the reappearance of plague and other infectious diseases as a result of overuse of antibiotics and other medicines, human settlement of previously uninhabited areas, international travel, and poverty. The fact that Western societies rarely encounter these diseases should not make us feel immune to their social, economic, cultural and human cost. Occasionally an outbreak occurs in the West, for example in Seattle in the early 1980s, when people ate tainted tofu which had not been pasteurized. Commercial tofu in sealed packaging should not be a cause for concern.

Smallpox has been officially eradicated through extensive worldwide immunization, although its course has probably influenced world history to a largely unappreciated degree. Blood Type O is especially susceptible to smallpox, which probably explains why the Native American population was decimated by the disease when it first came into contact with the Type A and B European settlers who carried it. Native Americans are almost 100 per cent Type O.

Typhoid, a common infection in areas of diminished hygiene or times of war, usually infects the blood and digestive tract. Type O is most susceptible to typhoid infection. Typhoid also shows a connection to the Rh blood groups, being found more frequently in Rh− individuals.

It is claimed that the *Anopheles* mosquito, which carries malaria, tends to bite Type B and Type O in preference to Type A and Type AB, although the common mosquito seems to prefer Type A and Type AB. Malaria is, again, an unfamiliar disease to the Western world, yet its global impact is tremendous.

According to the World Health Organization, more than 2.1 million people contract malaria every year.

Polio and viral meningitis

Polio, a viral infection of the nervous system, shows a higher frequency in Type B, which is more susceptible to virally-sparked nervous system disorders. Polio was epidemic and caused most cases of juvenile paralysis before the discovery of the Salk and Sabin vaccines.

Viral meningitis, an increasingly frequent and serious infection of the nervous system, is significantly more common in Type O than in other blood types, probably due to the Type O weakness against aggressive infections. Be alert to symptoms of fatigue, high fever, and a characteristic of meningitis called nuchal rigidity, a stiffness in the muscles of the neck.

Sinus infections

Type O and Type B are also typically more prone to chronic sinus infections. Very often, their doctors will prescribe an almost continuous supply of antibiotics, which banish the problem temporarily. But the sinus infections inevitably return, prompting the use of more antibiotics and, finally, surgery.

I have found that the herb collinsonia (stone root), which is used to treat swelling problems, like varicose veins, also helps sinusitis – perhaps because chronic sinusitis is a sort of haemorrhoid or varicose vein of the head. When I prescribe this herb to my patients with chronic sinusitis, the results are often astounding. Many of these patients no longer need antibiotics to treat their infections because the collinsonia removed the cause of the problem – swelling of the sinus tissue. If you have sinus problems, you may wish to try this herb. Collinsonia is not easy to find, but many of the larger health food shops carry it in a liquid tincture form. A typical dose is 20–25 drops in warm water taken orally 2–3 times daily. Do not worry about toxicity; this is a safe herb.

Occasionally a Type A or Type AB will develop sinusitis, although this is almost always the result of a high mucus-forming diet. Sinusitis in Type As usually responds well to diet changes alone.

Parasites (amoebic dysentery, *Giardia*, tapeworm and ascaris)

Given enough of a head start, parasites can live fairly well in anyone's digestive tract. Generally, however, they seem to have a special preference for Type A and Type AB digestive tracts, usually mimicking the Type A blood antigen to avoid detection. For example, the common amoeba parasite shows a preference for Type A and Type AB. In addition, it appears that Type A and Type AB are more prone to complications if amoebic cysts lodge in the liver. Type A and Type AB with amoebic dysentery should adopt strong measures to deal with the infection before it has a chance to migrate deeper into their bodies.

Blood Type A and Type AB are also sitting ducks for a common water contaminant, the parasite *Giardia lamblia*, more famously known as Montezuma's Revenge. This clever parasite mimics the appearance of Type A, which allows it entry into the Type A and Type AB immune systems, then quickly into the intestines. Type A and Type AB travellers should equip themselves with the herb golden seal to help stave off infection. Type As and Type ABs who drink from a water well should also be on the alert for the *Giardia lamblia* parasite.

Many of the parasitic worms, such as the tapeworm and the ascaris parasite, have a resemblance to Type A and Type B, and are found in greater frequency in people with these blood types. Because Type AB carries both A-like and B-like characteristics, they are particularly susceptible.

Tuberculosis and sarcoidosis

Tuberculosis was once considered almost completely eradicated from Western industrialized society, although it has now become more common. This is largely due to the high incidence of the disease in people with AIDS, and the homeless. An opportunistic infection, tuberculosis thrives in immune systems that have been weakened by poor hygiene and chronic disease. Tuberculosis of the lungs (pulmonary tuberculosis) is more common in Type O, whereas tuberculosis in other parts of the body shows a higher frequency in Type A.

Sarcoidosis, or sarcoid, is an inflammatory condition of the lungs and connective tissue which may actually be a form of immune reaction to tuberculosis. It was once thought to be much more common in African Americans compared with the general population, but in recent times it is being diagnosed more frequently in Caucasians, especially women. It shows a higher frequency of Type A over Type O.

Rh− individuals seem to be more susceptible to both tuberculosis and sarcoidosis.

Syphilis and urinary tract infections

Blood Type As seem to be more susceptible to venereal disease and syphilis, and often contract a more virulent strain. This is yet another reason to practise safe sex, especially if you are Type A.

There is good evidence that if you are Type B or Type AB, you are more susceptible to recurrent bladder infections (cystisis). That's because the most common bacteria-producing infections, such as *E. coli*, *Pseudomonas* and *Klebsiella*, possess a B-like appearance, and Type B and Type AB produce no anti-B antibodies.

Type Bs also have higher rates of kidney infections, called pyelonephritis. This is especially true of Type B non-secretors. If you are Type B and suffer from recurrent urinary problems, try to drink one or two glasses of a mixture of cranberry and pineapple juice every day.

LIVER DISEASE

Alcoholism-related liver disease

Alcoholism affects many bodily systems, but perhaps its most dramatic impact is on the liver. The 20 per cent of the population who are non-secretors (see Appendix E) seem to be the most prone to alcoholism, but their susceptibility has little to do with their secretor status. In an unfortunate and possibly random cellular twist, the gene which determines whether you're a non-secretor is located on the same part of the DNA as the gene for alcoholism. My patients who type as non-secretors always have an extensive family history of alcoholism.

Oddly enough, it is also non-secretors who seem to derive the most benefit to their hearts from a moderate intake of alcohol. A Danish study showing non-secretors to be a higher risk for ischaemic heart disease (a lack of blood flow into the arteries) theorized that a moderate consumption of alcohol altered the rate of insulin flow, slowing the accumulation of fats in the blood vessels. This conflicting message is hard to decipher.

The answer is probably that decisions about the role of alcohol should be made on an individual basis and with consideration for your blood type. From the standpoint of the effects of alcohol on the digestive and immune systems, none of the blood type diets allow spirits.

It is also clear that alcoholism has a major stress component. A Japanese research team discovered that a greater number of blood Type As received treatment for alcoholism than Type O or Type B. It is thought that Type As may have a predilection for seeking relaxation from stress by the ingestion of inhibition-releasing chemicals. It is certainly well documented that man has a long history of using intoxicants for pleasure, for pain, for transport to other realms, and for medicine.

Only about 3 per cent of the alcohol you consume passes through your body and is excreted. The rest is metabolized by the liver and processed in the stomach and small intestines. Over time, with heavy and regular consumption, the liver begins to deteriorate. The end result can be cirrhosis of the liver, severe malnutrition from mal-absorption of foods, and ultimately death.

Gallstones, cirrhosis and jaundice

Of course, not all liver disease is linked to alcohol. Infections, allergies, and metabolic disorders can all cause liver damage. For example, jaundice, or yellowing of the skin, is often seen in people with hepatitis, and gallstones have been linked to obesity. Cirrhosis can be caused by infections, diseases of the bile ducts, or other illnesses that affect the liver.

For reasons we do not fully understand, Type As, Type Bs

and Type ABs tend to have higher levels of gallstones, diseases of the bile ducts, jaundice and cirrhosis of the liver than Type Os. Type As have the highest levels and are also reported to be the most susceptible to pancreatic tumours.

Liver flukes and other tropical infections
Common tropical infections of the liver causing fibrosis or scarring appear to a marked degree more frequently in Type As – and to a lesser extent in Type B and Type AB. Type O, which may have developed anti-A and anti-B antibodies as an early protection against these parasites, is relatively immune to them.

My office has successfully treated many cases of liver disease using many of the herbal compounds discussed in Chapter 10. In most cases, the patients who develop liver disease are Type A and Type B, non-secretors.

* * *

Case history: Liver disease
Gerard, 38: Type B

Gerard was a 38-year-old man with a history of sclerosing cholangitis, an inflammatory condition of the liver's bile ducts, causing scarring. Usually this condition leads to the necessity of a liver transplant. When I first saw Gerard in July 1994, he was jaundiced and had horrible pruritus (itching) from deposits of bilirubin, an orange-yellow bile pigment, in his skin. Because of this condition, his cholesterol was also elevated to 325. Gerard's serum bile acids were over 2000 (normal is under 100), he had a bilirubin level of 4.1 (normal is under 1) and all his liver enzymes were sharply elevated, indicating extensive damage to his liver tissue. Gerard was a pretty shrewd man, who knew what his chances were, and frankly, he was preparing to die.

I started Gerard on the basic Type B diet and a botanical protocol of liver-specific antioxidants. These are antioxidants that preferentially deposit in the liver instead of in other organs. Gerard did very well in the intervening year, having only one flare-up of itching and jaundice.

Recently Gerard underwent surgery to remove his gall-bladder. When the surgeon examined his liver and major bile ducts, she later told him that they looked normal, although the tissue around his bile ducts was a little thinner than usual.

Case History: Cirrhosis
Estel, 67: Type A

Estel was a 67-year-old woman who first came to my office in October 1991 for an inflammatory condition of the the liver called primary biliary cirrhosis which results in destruction of the liver. Most cases eventually go on to have a liver transplant.

Estel admitted that she was once a heavy drinker, but no longer. Her condition was probably linked to a lifetime of alcohol consumption, even though she may not have even been an alcoholic, in the strictest sense. Three or four drinks a day, every day, for 40 years can lead to cirrhosis.

Estel's liver enzymes were markedly elevated: the alkaline phosphatase, for example, was in the high 800s (normal is under 60). Since she was a Type A non-secretor, I immediately put her on the Type A diet and a protocol of liver-specific antioxidants. Estel began to show results almost immediately, and her condition continued to improve.

By September 1992, almost a year after her first visit, Estel's alkaline phosphatase had dropped to 500.

Although her liver has shown no signs of further deterioration since that time, Estel developed swelling of the veins around her oesophagus, a common condition in people with liver disease, and this was treated successfully. She continues to do well and shows no sign of requiring liver transplantion.

Case History: Liver deterioration
Sandra, 70: Type A

Sandra arrived in my office in January 1993, suffering from a liver condition that was difficult to determine. All of her liver enzymes were elevated, and she also had a condition called ascites which meant swelling and an extensive amount of fluid being retained in her abdomen. Ascites is common in many cases of advanced liver failure. Sandra's specialist was not treating her liver deterioration, probably expecting her to eventually require a transplant. He was prescribing diuretics to help remove the fluid from her abdomen, but the diuretics were causing her to lose large amounts of potassium, which probably accounted for her overwhelming fatigue.

I prescribed the Type A diet with liver-specific botanicals. Within four months, all evidence of Sandra's fluid retention disappeared, and the liver enzymes returned to normal. Sandra was initially quite anaemic – with a haematocrit of 27.1 where normal for a woman is over 38. By February 1994 her haematocrit had risen to 40.8. She continues to be asymptomatic.

* * *

SKIN DISORDERS

To date, there is little blood type-specific information available on skin disorders. We do know, however, that conditions like dermatisis and psoriasis usually result from allergic chemicals acting within the blood. It is worth noting again that many of the common food lectins specific for one blood type or another can interact with the blood and digestive tissues, causing the liberation of histamine and other inflammatory chemicals.

Allergic skin reactions to chemicals or abrasives show the highest incidences in Type A and Type AB. Psoriasis is found more frequently in Type Os. My own experience is that many Type Os who develop psoriasis have diets that are too high in grains or dairy products.

* * *

Case History: Psoriasis
(From Dr Anne Marie Lambert ND, Honolulu, Hawaii)
Mariel, 66: Type 0

My colleague, Dr Lambert, used my blood type protocol to treat a complicated case of psoriasis in an older woman.

Mariel went to see Dr Lambert in March 1994. Her symptoms included: severe shortness of breath, difficulty walking (with limited range of motion in all joints), psoriasis lesions covering 70 per cent of her skin surface, and burning pain throughout her body, especially in her muscles and joints. Her medical history was a catalogue of constant medical problems: vaginal/bowel repairs (1944–5), appendectomy (1949), hysterectomy (1974), history of ovarian cysts, psoriasis (1978), hospitalization for pneumonia (1987), psoriatic arthritis (1991), and osteoporosis (1992).

Mariel told Dr Lambert that her typical diet was high in dairy, wheat, corn, nuts and processed foods, with a high sugar and fat content. She said that she craved sweets, nuts and bananas. This was a terrible diet for almost anyone, but it was anathema to someone of Muriel's blood type.

Dr Lambert immediately started Mariel on a moderated Type O diet, which initially excluded red meat and nuts, and with additional vitamins and minerals. Within two months, there was a marked decrease in the swelling of Mariel's joints, improved breathing, and her psoriatic lesions were healing. By June, Mariel's psoriasis covered only 20 per cent of her body, and the lesions were nearly healed. There was a marked improvement in her breathing, her pain had lessened by half, and the range of motion in her joints continued to improve. By July, Mariel's psoriasis was no longer evident, there was only slight swelling in the joint spaces, and her breathing was no longer laboured.

At a follow-up visit to Dr Lambert on 10 October 1994, Mariel's breathing had improved, and she had no new lesions on her skin.

Mariel had been to numerous medical professionals since she became ill. She had tried all types of conventional as well as alternative therapies, including food plans specifically designed for psoriatic arthritis and asthma. Although these diets were well intended, none of them were specifically tailored to ensure compatibility with Mariel's blood. The Type O diet was able to provide nutrition without causing health problems from foods that were incompatible with Mariel's blood. With the exception of some minor pain relief from Chinese herbs, none of the other treatments had been successful. Mariel considered her progress a miracle!

* * *

WOMEN/REPRODUCTION

Pregnancy and infertility
Many of the disorders related to pregnancy result from some form of blood type incompatibility – either between the mother and the foetus, or between the mother and the father. Unfortunately, we only have initial studies on this phenomenon, and have little idea about its ultimate implications. I suggest that you read this section in the spirit of information-gathering, not hysteria. Sometimes a little bit of knowledge can be dangerous unless you keep it in perspective.

Toxaemia of pregnancy
As early as 1905 it was proposed that some form of blood type sensitization resulted in pregnancy toxaemia – a poisoning of the blood that can occur in late pregnancy and cause grave illness and even death. In a later study, an excess of Type O women were found to suffer from toxaemia, possibly resulting from a reaction to a Type A or Type B foetus.

Birth defects
Blood type incompatibility, which may occur between a Type O mother and a Type A father, has been implicated in several common birth defects, including hydatiform mole, choriocarcinoma, spina bifida and anencephaly. Several studies imply that these disorders appear to be maternal ABO incompatibility with foetal nervous and blood tissue.

Haemolytic disease of the newborn
Haemolytic (blood destroying) disease of the newborn is the primary condition related to the positive/negative aspect of your blood. It is a condition that only afflicts the offspring of

Rh− women, so if you are O, A, B, or AB positive, it doesn't concern you.

Some 50 years ago, researchers discovered that Rh− women who were missing an antigen and were carrying Rh+ babies had a unique situation. The Rh+ babies carried the Rh antigen on their blood cells. Unlike the major blood type system where the antibodies to other blood types develop from birth, Rh− people do not make an antibody to the Rh antigen unless they are first sensitized. This sensitization usually occurs when blood is exchanged between the mother and infant during birth, so the mother's immune system does not have enough time to react to the first baby, and that baby suffers no consequences. However, should a subsequent conception result in another Rh+ baby, the mother, now sensitized, will produce anitbodies to the baby's blood type, potentially causing birth defects and even infant death. Fortunately, there is a vaccine for this condition which is given to Rh− women after the birth of their first child, and after every subsequent birth. This problem shouldn't arise, but it's best to know your Rh status so you can be certain that the vaccine is administered.

Infertility and habitual miscarriage

For 40 years, scientists have been studying the reasons why childlessness seems to more common among Type A, Type B, and Type AB women than Type O women. Many researchers have suggested that infertility and habitual abortion may be the result of antibodies in a woman's vaginal secretions reacting with blood type antigens on her husband's sperm. A 1975 study of 288 miscarried foetuses showed that there were a predominance of Type A, Type B and Type AB foetuses, which may have been the result of incompatibility with Type O mothers and their anti-A and anti-B antibodies.

A large sample of families showed that the rate of miscarriages were highest when the mother and father were ABO incompatible, such as a Type O mother and Type A father. In Caucasian and African mothers, Type B foetuses that were incompatible with the mother's Type O or Type A blood, were more frequently involved in miscarriages.

This link to infertility is not yet fully established. In my own practice, I find that there are many reasons for fertility problems, including food allergies, poor diet, obesity, and stress.

* * *

Case History: Repeated miscarriage
Lana, 42: Type A

Lana came to my office in September 1993 after a long history of repeated miscarriages. She told me she'd heard about me from someone she had been talking to in the waiting room of her fertility doctor. Lana was desperate. In the previous 10 years she'd had over 20 miscarriages, and she was just about to give up on trying to start a family. I suggested that she try the Type A diet. For the next year, Lana followed the blood type diet assiduously, also taking several botanical preparations to strengthen the muscular tone of her uterus. At the end of the year, she became pregnant. She was thrilled, but also very nervous. Now, in addition to her previous miscarriages, Lana was worried about her age and the possibility of the foetus having Down's syndrome. Her obstetrician recommended amniocentesis, which is common for women over 40, but I advised against it because the procedure carries a risk of miscarriage. After talking with her husband, Lana decided to forgo the amniocentesis, accepting the possibility of a birth defect. In January 1995, she delivered a perfectly healthy baby boy.

Case History: Infertility
Nieves, 44: Type B

Nieves, a 44-year-old South American massage therapist, first came to see me in 1991 for a variety of digestive problems. Most of her digestive complaints were resolved within one year of following the Type B diet.

One day Nieves shyly announced that she was pregnant. Although she had not told me before, she now said that she and her husband had tried for many years to conceive a child, but had finally given up hope. She believed that the Type B diet was responsible for restoring her fertility. Approximately nine months later, Nieves delivered a healthy baby girl. They named her Nasha, meaning 'gift from God'.

Note: Sex ratios

In both European and non-European populations, the rate of male offspring is higher in Type O babies born to Type O mothers. This is also true if the baby and mother are both Type B. The opposite is true of Type A babies to Type A mothers, where female offspring are more frequent.

Menopause and menstrual problems

Menopause affects every mid-life woman regardless of her blood type. A decrease in oestrogen and progesterone, the two basic female hormones, causes profound mental and physical problems for many women, including hot flushes, loss of libido, depression, hair loss and skin changes.

The decline in female hormones also creates a risk of cardiovascular disease, as it appears that oestrogen provides protection to the heart and lowers cholesterol levels. Osteoporosis, a thinning of the bones that leads to frailty and even death, is another outcome of oestrogen deficiency.

With our new-found understanding of the risks associated with hormone depletion, many doctors prescribe hormone replacement therapy, involving high doses of oestrogen and sometimes progesterone. Many woman are concerned about conventional oestrogen replacement therapy because some studies show a greater risk of breast cancer in women who use these hormones – primarily when there is a family of breast cancer. The question of whether or not to take these synthetic hormones is a confusing dilemma.

Knowing your blood type can begin to resolve the conflict and help you decide which approach is best for your own personal needs.

If you are Type O or Type B and entering the menopause, begin to exercise in a manner recommended for your blood type, and in a way appropriate to your current state of fitness and lifestyle. Eat a high protein diet. Conventional oestrogen replacement generally works reasonably well for Type O and Type B women, unless you have high-risk factors for breast cancer.

If you are Type A or Type AB, you should avoid using conventional oestrogen replacement, because of your unusually high susceptibility to breast cancer (See chapter 10). Instead, use the newly available phyto-oestrogens, which are oestrogen- and progesterone-like preparations derived from plants, principally soya beans, alfalfa and yams. Many of these preparations are available as a cream which can be applied to the skin several times a day. Plant phyto-oestrogens are typically high in the oestrogen fraction called oestriol, whereas chemical oestrogens are based on oestradiol. The medical literature conclusively shows that supplementation with oestriol inhibits the occurrence of breast cancer.

Phyto-oestrogens lack the potency of the chemical oestrogens, but they are definitely effective against many of the troubling symptoms of menopause, including hot flushes and vaginal dryness. Because they are only weak oestrogens, they will not suppress any oestrogen production by the body, unlike the chemical oestrogen. For the woman who is not taking any oestrogen supplementation because of a family history of breast cancer, the phyto-oestrogens are a godsend.

Talk to your gynaecologist about using these preparations. If you have none of the risk factors for breast cancer, the stronger chemical oestrogen is more effective for reducing heart disease and osteoporosis, in addition to the symptoms of menopause.

It is interesting that in Japan, where the typical diet is high in phyto-oestrogens, there is no concise word for menopause. Undoubtedly the widespread use of soya products, which contain the phyto-oestrogens genestein and diaziden, serves to modulate the severe symptoms of the menopause.

* * *

Case History: Menstrual problems
Patty, 45: Type O

Patty was a 45-year-old African American woman with a variety of problems including arthritis, high blood pressure and severe pre-mentrual syndrome (PMS/PMT) with heavy bleeding. I first met Patty in December 1994 when she came to my office accompanied by her husband. At the time, she was being treated by one drug or another for her ailments. I learned that Patty had been consuming a basically vegetarian diet, so it was no surprise that she was also anaemic. I recommended that she begin exercising, adopt the Type O high-protein diet, and I prescribed a course of botanical medicines.

Within two months, Patty made an astounding turn-about. Her arthritis was cured, the hypertension under control and the last two months had been free of PMS. Her menstrual flow was now normal.

* * *

I wish it were possible to supply you with a more detailed and complete list of diseases. Perhaps then we could more fully estimate their link to blood type.

The cause and effect of disease often crosses all boundaries. Cancer, for instance, seems to snatch at both the young and old thoughtlessly and without regard to circumstance or exposure.

It is clear, however, that there are many diseases that show a strong propensity for a specific blood type. I hope the evidence I've offered in this discussion of blood type and disease has proved this relationship.

If nothing else, knowing your chances, assessing your risk factors, and understanding the situation gives you another way to take positive action against the forces that may often leave you feeling you have no control.

10

Blood Type and Cancer: The Fight To Heal

I EXPERIENCE A PARTICULAR SURGE of passion whenever I examine the healing connection between blood type and cancer. My mother died of breast cancer 10 years ago, after an agonizing experience.

My mother was a wonderful woman, whose simple Spanish values guarded us all against any pretence or pomp. She was an anomaly in our family – a Type A who ate what she chose to eat. She had the notorious Corsican strong will. In her house (my parents were divorced), she served a basic Mediterranean diet of meats and salads and some processed foods. In spite of my father's blood type work, there wasn't a soya bean in sight when we stayed with Mother.

Anyone who has seen a family member or friend engage in a valiant but ultimately fruitless struggle against cancer, knows that there is nothing quite so heartbreaking. Watching my mother as she went from mastectomy to chemotherapy, from a brief remission to recurrence, I could almost visualize the armies of invisible invaders, stealing their way into her healthy cells and gaining a strong foothold before sweeping through her immune system like barbarians waging a surprise attack. In the end, nothing could be done to stop them. They won.

In the years since my mother's death, I have found myself returning again and again to the mysteries of cancer. I have often wondered if my mother might have been spared had she adhered to a Type A diet, or if she was somehow genetically predetermined to fight and lose this battle. I have dedicated myself to finding those answers on her behalf. You might say I have a Corsican-style vendetta against breast cancer above all other cancers.

Does cancer find an inherently more fertile ground to grow and develop in the body of one blood type than in another? The answer is a certain 'yes'.

There is undeniable evidence that persons with Type A or Type AB blood have an overall higher rate of cancer and poorer odds of survival than Type O and Type B. Actually, as early as the 1940s, the American Medical Association stated that Type AB had the greatest rate of cancer of all the blood types, but the news didn't make headlines, probably because Type ABs constitute such a low percentage of the population. Statistically, their high cancer rate didn't cause the same kind of alarm as the information about the more common Type A. But from a personal standpoint, that's surely of little comfort to the individuals with Type AB blood. Researchers may treat cancer like a numbers game; I prefer to treat it as a personal crisis in the life of a single individual.

Type O and Type B show a much lower incidence of cancer, but we don't yet have enough information to say exactly why that is. There are important clues we can explore, however, in the antigen and antibody activity of the different blood types.

Having said that, the blood type–cancer connection is highly complex and in many ways mysterious. Be clear that being Type AB or Type A doesn't mean that it's certain or even likely that you personally are going to get cancer, any more than being Type O or Type B means you'll be absolutely spared. There are many causes of cancer, and we are still haunted by the mystery of why people with no evident risk factors contract the disease.

Increasingly, blood type has emerged as a vital factor, but it is only one piece of the puzzle. There are many causes of cancer – chemical carcinogens, radiation and genetics, to name a few. These factors are largely independent of blood type, and as such would not produce enough of a difference in the population to be able to be predicted on the basis of blood type. For example, cigarette smoking could easily mask or weaken a blood type association because it is a powerful enough carcinogen to cause cancer all by itself – regardless of your inherent susceptibility or lack of it.

There is an enormous amount of scientific research on the molecular relationship between blood type and cancer. But the research has practically ignored the question of whether a person with one blood type or another has a better chance of surviving particular cancers.

Who lives and who dies? Who survives and who doesn't? This, in my opinion, is the great missing link in the research on cancer and blood type. The real blood type–cancer connection resides in the rates of resolution rather than in the rates of occurrence among the different blood types. And that connection may be the glue of lectins.

The cancer-lectin connection

Shakespeare once wrote that 'There is some soul of goodness in things evil.' In some instances, like chemotherapy treatments to fight cancer, it is expedient and even beneficial to use a poison. In relationship to cancer, lectins serve two purposes: They can be used to agglutinate cancerous cells, and thus act as a catalyst for the immune system – a wake-up call to get busy and protect the good cells.

How does this happen? Under normal circumstances, the production of surface sugars by a cell is highly specific and controlled. Not in a cancer cell. Because the genetic material is scrambled, cancer cells lose control over the production of their surface sugars, and usually manufacture them in greater amounts than a normal cell would. Cancer cells are more liable to tangle up if they come in contact with the appropriate lectin.

Malignant cancerous cells are as much as 100 times more sensitive to the agglutinating effects of lectins than normal cells. If two slides are prepared, one containing normal cells and the other malignant, an equal dose of the appropriate lectin will convert the slide with malignant cells into a huge entangled clump, whereas the slide of normal cells will show little, if any, change.

When malignant cells become agglutinated into huge tangles of hundreds, thousands or millions of cancer cells, the immune

The Lectin-Cancer Connection

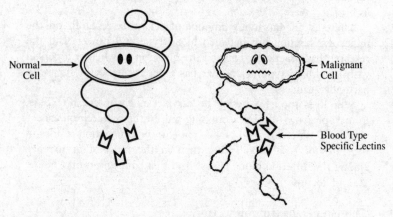

Normal Cell

Malignant Cell

Blood Type Specific Lectins

Why lectins agglutinate cancer cells. The cells depicted on the left side of the drawing represent non-malignant cells. Because the production of surface sugars is controlled by intact genetic material, normal cell walls have surface sugars arranged in an orderly pattern. But malignant cells have many more surface sugars because their genetic material is flawed, resulting in the malignant cell producing uncontrolled amounts of these sugars. If a blood type–specific food lectin is added to a suspension of normal and malignant cells, it will interact more aggressively with the "fuzzier" malignant cells than with the "smoother" normal cells.

system becomes reactivated. Now the antibodies can target the clumps of cancer cells, identifying them for destruction. This search-and-destroy mission is usually carried out by powerful scavenger cells found in the liver.

If you were to go into a medical database and key in 'lectins' and 'cancer', the printer would be working overtime for days. Lectins are extensively used to study the molecular biology of cancer because they make excellent probes, helping to identify unique antigens called markers on the surface of the cancer cells. Beyond this, their use is limited, which is unfortunate because they are so ubiquitous in common foods. By identifying the blood type of a person with a particular cancer, and using the appropriate lectins derived from the Blood Type Plan, a powerful new tool can be utilized by any cancer patient to improve their odds of survival.

Enter the blood type

An enormous amount of cell division occurs in the course of one's lifetime. Given these odds, it is amazing that cancer doesn't occur more often. This is probably because the immune system has a special ability to detect and eliminate the vast majority of mutations that take place on a day-to-day basis. Cancer probably results from a breakdown in this surveillance, the successful cancer cell tricking the immune system into impotency by mimicking normal cells. As we have already seen, the blood types possess unique powers of surveillance, depending on the shape and form of the intruder.

This gives you a rough idea of how blood types, agglutinating lectins, and cancer interact together. The obvious next question is: what does it mean? And if you are personally worried about cancer, what does this mean for you?

To date, the only cancer for which we have substantial information about the blood type connection is breast cancer. I will talk about it in some detail. The other cancers are less well defined regarding blood types, but we do have limited information that I will share. We also know that there are many food-related links that undoubtedly apply to all, or most cancers, and we'll study these carefully in view of our knowledge about nutrition and blood types. There are also some innovative naturopathic therapies that are held in high regard and are gaining wider favour.

The research goes on, but it is an agonizingly slow process. Even now, as I write this, I am beginning the eighth year of a ten-year trial on reproductive cancers, using the blood type diets. My results are encouraging. So far, the women in my trial have double the survival rate published by the American Cancer Society. By the time I release the results in another two years, I expect to make it scientifically demonstrable that the Blood Type Plan plays a role in cancer remission.

BREAST CANCER

A number of years ago, while taking histories on new patients, I began to notice that many women who had suffered from breast cancer at some time in their distant pasts, and had fully recovered, were Type Os or Type Bs. Their rate of recovery was especially impressive since most of them told me that their treatment had not been very aggressive – usually no more than surgical excision, only rarely including radiation or chemography.

How could this be? The statistics on breast cancer show that, even with the most aggressive treatment, only 19–25 per cent of women survive 5–10 years after the diagnosis. Yet these women had survived for a much longer time with only minimal therapy. Was it possible that being Type O or Type B helped to protect them against the spread of the disease or a recurrence?

Over the years, I also began to notice a distinct tendency in Type A women with breast cancer – and also in Type AB women, although I haven't seen many with that rare blood type – to suffer from a more aggressive malignancy and a lower survival rate, even when biopsies taken from the lymph nodes showed that they were free of cancer. Through my own clinical experience and study of scientific literature, I concluded that there is a major connection between surviving breast cancer and your blood type.

In 1991, a study appeared in the *Lancet*, an English medical journal, which may have provided part of the answer. Researchers reported that it appeared possible to predict whether or not a breast cancer would spread to the lymph nodes by virtue of its characteristics when treated with a stain containing a lectin from the edible snail, *Helix pomatia*. They reported a strong association between the uptake of the snail lectin and the subsequent development of metastasis (transfer of cancer) to the lymph nodes. In other words, antigens on the surface of the primary breast cancer cells were changing, and this change was allowing the cancer to spread into the lymph nodes. The key is that the lectin of *Helix pomatia* is highly specific – to Blood Type A.

The researchers studying breast cancer discovered that as the cancer cells changed, they made themselves more A-like. This allowed them to bypass all of the body's defences and rage unimpeded into the defenceless lymph.

Did my Type O patients survive because they were Type O? Did my Type B patients survive because they were Type B? It certainly looked that way.

There is a confirmation in our scientific understanding of

cancer. Many tumour cells have unique antigens, or markers, on their surfaces. For instance, breast cancer patients often show high levels of Cancer Antigen 15-3 (CA15-3), a marker for breast cancer. Ovarian cancer patients often have high levels of Cancer Antigen 125 (CA125), while prostate cancer patients can have an elevated Prostate Specific Antigen (PSA) and so on. These antigens are often used to track the progress of the disease and effectiveness of treatment, and are called tumour markers. Many tumour markers possess blood type activity. Sometimes the tumour markers are incomplete or corrupted blood type antigens, which in a normal cell would have gone on to form a part of the person's blood type system.

Not surprisingly, many of these tumour markers have A-like qualities, which allow them easy access to the Type A and Type AB systems. There they are welcomed as 'self' – the ultimate molecular Trojan Horse. Obviously, the A-like intruders would be more easily detected and eliminated if they were to slip into a Type O or Type B system.

Breast cancer markers are overwhelmingly A-like. This answers my question about the differing rates of recurrence in my patients. Although my Type O and Type B patients had developed breast cancer, their anti-A antigens were better able to fight it off, rounding up the early cancer cells and destroying them. On the other hand, my Type A and Type AB patients couldn't fight as well because they couldn't see their opponents. Everywhere they turned, the cells looked just like them – and they were unable to detect the mutated cancer cells beneath their clever masks.

* * *

Case History: Preventing breast cancer
Anne, 47: Type A

Four years ago Anne came to the office for a general check-up, without any real physical complaints. But while I was doing her medical history, I learned that Anne's family had a high incidence of breast cancer on both her mother's and father's sides – and the mortality rate among those who had the disease was very high.

Anne knew about her genetic risk factors, but she was surprised to learn that her Type A blood presented an additional risk factor. 'I don't suppose it makes any difference, though,' she said. 'Either I'm going to get breast cancer or I'm not. There's nothing I can really do about it.'

I advised Anne that there were several measures she could take. First, because of her family history, she needed to be extra vigilant about suspicious breast lumps, perform frequent breast self-examinations, and have routine mammograms.

'When was your last mammogram?' I asked. Anne sheepishly told me that her last mammogram had been seven years ago. It turned out that Anne was strongly disinclined to avail herself of any conventional medical techniques. She had educated herself about herbs and vitamins, and often used them effectively to treat herself. But when it came to more intrusive medical treatments, she shied away. However, she did promise to schedule a mammogram.

Anne's mammogram was clean, and she began a concentrated program of cancer avoidance. The Type A diet was an easy transition for Anne because she already ate a primarily vegetarian diet. I fine-tuned the diet with anti-cancer foods – especially increasing the amount of soya, and adding specific naturopathic herbs. Anne began to study yoga. She told me that for the first time in her adult life, she wasn't constantly worrying about cancer.

A year later, Anne had a second mammogram. This time a suspicious mark was detected in her left breast. A biopsy showed it to be a precancerous condition known as neoplasia. Essentially, neoplasia is the presence of mutated cells. It's not cancer, but it can become cancer if the cells continue to deteriorate and multiply. During the biopsy, Anne's doctor completely removed the pre-cancerous mark.

Three years later, there have been no new growths detected, although we are watching Anne very carefully. She continues to follow the Type A diet religiously, and says she has never felt healthier.

Of all the functions a physician can perform, none is more elegant and valuable than successful prediction and intervention. I was glad Anne came to me when she did, and that she took all the right steps.

* * *

THE ANTIGEN VACCINE
Breast cancer continues to be baffling and too often deadly. But there are some signs that blood type may represent a key to the cure.

Dr George Springer, a research scientist with the Bligh Cancer Center at the University of Chicago School of Medicine, has been investigating the effects of a vaccine whose basis is a molecule called the T antigen. Since the 1950s, Springer has been one of the most important investigators in the role of blood type in disease. His contributions to the field are phenomenal. His work on the T antigen has been most promising.

The T antigen is a common tumour marker found in many cancers, especially breast cancer. Healthy, cancer-free people carry antibodies against the T antigen, so it is never seen in them.

Springer believes that a vaccine composed of the T antigen and the tumour marker CA 15-3 can help jolt and then reawaken the suppressed immune systems of cancer patients, helping them to attack and destroy the cancerous cells. For the past 20 years, Springer and his colleagues have been using a vaccine derived from the T antigen as a long-term treatment against the recurrence of advanced breast cancer.

Although the study group is small – less than 25 women – the results are impressive. All of the 11 breast cancer patients with severely advanced disease (Stage III and Stage IV), survived for longer than five years – remarkable in what is considered end-stage cancer; while six of them (three Stage III and three Stage IV) survived for between 10–18 years. These results are nothing short of miraculous.

Springer's continued work on blood type systems and cancer convinces me that the natural evolution of our understanding of blood types will eventually provide not just information on risk factors, but also a cure for every manifestation of the disease.

OTHER FORMS OF CANCER

The pathology of this disease is fundamentally the same in all cancers. Yet there are variations related both to cause and to blood type. The A-like or B-like tumour markers exert remarkable control over the way the body's immune system reacts to the cancer's invasion and growth.

Again, almost all cancers show a preference for Type A and Type AB, although there are occasional forms that are B-like – such as female reproductive and bladder cancers. Type Os seem to be far more resistant to developing almost any cancer. Intolerant and hostile, I believe that the more simple fucose sugars of Type Os dispose them to tossing off the A-like – or in some cases B-like – cancer cells, and developing anti-A or anti-B antibodies.

Again, we unfortunately know little about the full implications of the blood type link in cancers other than breast cancer. However, it most likely follows a similar course. Let's examine some of the most common forms of cancer.

Brain tumours

Most cancers of the brain and nervous system, such as glioma multiforma and astrocytoma, show a preference for Type A and Type AB. Their tumour markers are A-like.

Female reproductive cancers

Cancers of the female reproductive system (uterine, cervical, ovarian, and labial) show a preference for Type A and Type AB women. However, there are also a high number of Type B women who suffer from these cancers. This implies that there are different tumour markers created, depending upon the circumstances. Ovarian cysts and uterine fibroids, which are usually benign but may be a sign of susceptibility to cancer, generate copious amounts of Type A and Type B antigens.

As I mentioned earlier, I am currently in the eighth year of a ten year clinical trial of women with reproductive cancer. Most of my patients are Type A, and a few are Type B. Only occasionally do I treat a Type AB woman, but that is also because there aren't very many of them.

Colon cancer

Blood type is not the strongest determinant for the various forms of colon cancer. The real risk factors for the conditions that lead to colon cancer are related to diet, lifestyle and temperament. Ulcerative colitis, Crohn's Disease, and irritable bowel syndrome left unmitigated eventually leave the system depleted and open to cancer. A high-fat diet, combined with smoking and alcohol consumption, create the ideal environment for digestive cancers. The risk is greater if you have a family history of colon cancer.

Mouth and upper digestive cancers

Cancers of the lip, tongue, gums and cheek; tumours of the salivary gland; oesophageal cancer – are all strongly linked to Type A and Type AB. Most of these cancers are self-generated, in that the risks can be minimized if you abstain from tobacco, moderate your alcoholic consumption, and watch your diet.

Stomach and oesophageal cancer

Stomach cancer is attracted to low levels of stomach acid, a Type A and Type AB trait. In well over 63,000 cases of stomach cancer studied, Type A and Type AB were predominant.

Stomach cancer is epidemic in China, Japan, and Korea because the typical diet is rich in smoked, pickled, and fermented foods. These Asian dietary staples seem to counter any of the good that soya beans might do, perhaps because they are packed with carcinogenic nitrates. Asian Type Bs, who have higher levels of stomach acid, aren't as prone to stomach cancer, even if they eat some of the same foods.

Pancreatic, liver, gall-bladder and bile duct cancers

These cancers are rare in Type Os, with their hardy digestive systems. Type A and Type AB are at most risk, with Type Bs having some susceptibility – especially if they consume many 'harsh' foods like nuts and seeds.

Several of the earlier therapies for these cancers included large portions of fresh liver from sheep, horse, and buffalo. They seemed to help, but no one knew why. It was later discovered that the livers contained lectins that slowed the growth and spread of pancreative, gall-bladder, and bile duct cancers.

* * *

Case History: Liver cancer
Cathy, 49: Type A

Cathy first sought medical attention in the late 1980s for a suspicious growth in her abdomen which turned out to be an aggressive form of liver cancer. She was treated at Harvard's Deaconess Hospital in Boston, Massachusetts, and eventually received a liver transplant. She was referred to me in 1990.

In the subsequent two years, most of my focus was on using naturopathic techniques to replace the immuno-suppressing anti-rejection drugs needed to help her keep her transplanted liver. Cathy's condition improved to the point where she was able to stop her drug therapy.

However, in 1992, Cathy noticed some shortness of breath, and at her check-up at Harvard, doctors noticed suspicious lesions on her chest X-ray. These turned out to be cancer.

Cathy and her doctors were on the horns of a dilemma. Her lungs were so heavily laced with cancer, surgery was out of the question ('It would be like picking cherries' said her surgeon), and her liver transplant ruled out chemotherapy.

We went to work, using the basic type A-lectin cancer diet and other immune-enhancing botanicals. I also recommended a preparation made from shark cartilage for Cathy to take orally and use as an enema.

In an amazing series of correspondences, Cathy's surgical team at Harvard kept me up to date on her progress. In a letter dated 3 September 1992, I was informed that the lesions in Cathy's lung had shrunk and looked more like scar tissue. Subsequent letters confirmed these findings. By 1993, even the scar tissue had begun to disappear.

Cathy was stunned and overjoyed. 'When they told me that the cancer seemed to be going into remission, I felt as if I had won the lottery,' she said happily. Cathy went on to live three symptom-free years. Unfortunately, her cancer returned at that point, and she later died.

The case is especially interesting for two reasons. First, throughout this time Cathy received no treatment other than naturopathic. Second, her team at Harvard was open-minded and supportive of her using a naturopathic doctor. Perhaps what we have seen here is a tiny glimpse of the future – all medical systems working together for the betterment of the patient.

Also, the total cost of Cathy's naturopathic therapy was less than $1500, as opposed to the tens of thousands she might have spent on conventional treatment.

* * *

Lung cancer

Lung cancer is truly non-specific. It is one of the few cancers which has no particular blood type connection. Lung cancer is most commonly caused by cigarette smoking.

Lung cancer *is* caused by many other things as well. There are people who have never smoked who will die of lung cancer as you are reading this sentence. But we all know that smoking is the overwhelming cause of lung cancer. Tobacco is such a powerful carcinogen in its own right that it bypasses anything so obvious, so ordered, as predilection.

Lymphomas, leukaemias, and Hodgkin's Disease

This is a form of cancer to which Type Os are predisposed – maybe. Although these cancers of the blood and lymph preferentially afflict Type Os, they may not be true cancers at all, but rather viral infections that have run amok. This would make some sense in light of what we know about Type Os; they're actually pretty good at fighting most cancers, but the Type O antigen is not well designed for fighting viruses.

Prostate cancer

There appears to be a higher level of prostate cancer in secretors (see Appendix E). My own experience has been that a greater number of Type A and Type AB men suffer from prostate cancer than do Type O or Type B men. A type A or Type AB secretor is at the highest risk.

Skin and bone cancers

Skin cancers are unique in that there are a greater number of Type Os who suffer from them. Perhaps the lighter skins of northern Europeans – who are predominantly Type Os – are reacting to the increasing levels of ultraviolet radiation caused by environmental pollution.

Malignant melanoma is the deadliest form of skin cancer. Type A and Type AB are at greatest risk for this condition, although Type O and Type B are not immune.

Bone cancers seem to show a consistent preference for Type B, although there is some risk for Type A and Type AB.

Urinary tract cancer

Bladder cancer in both men and women occurs most often in Type A and Type B. Type ABs, who have the double measure of both A and B characteristics, are probably at the greatest risk of all.

Far more than Type As, Type Bs who suffer from recurrent bladder and kidney infection should be especially careful with the management of this problem, as it inevitably leads to more serious disease.

One puzzling connection that is yet to be unravelled: wheatgerm agglutinin, the lectin that can act favourably against both lobular and intraductal breast cancers, paradoxically accelerates the growth of bladder cancer cells.

FIGHTING BACK

Cancer always seems to present a discouraging picture. I imagine that if you are Type A or Type AB, you may be thinking grim thoughts. Remember though that susceptibility is a single factor among many. I believe that knowing your predilection for cancer, and understanding the workings of your specific blood type, gives you more opportunity to fight back. The following strategies can give you a way to make a difference for yourself, especially if you are Type A or Type AB. In particular, many of the foods suggested are tailored for these blood types. Current research has primarily focused on the A-like markers for breast cancer, and little investigation has been conducted regarding the B-like cancers. Unfortunately, this means that while the cancer-fighting foods suggested here may be very effective for Type As and Type ABs, they won't necessarily help Type Bs or Type Os. In fact, most of these foods (peanuts, lentils, and wheatgerm) cause other problems for these two blood types.

The clinical trials I am currently conducting, along with the work of other scientists and researchers, will one day give us a deeper understanding of the cancer-diet connection for all the blood types. In the meantime, Type Bs and Type Os can reduce the chance of the cell mutations that can lead to cancer by adhering to their blood type diet. If you already have a cancerous condition, take special note of the other therapies in this section, especially the pneumococcus vaccine. Further research will offer a more complete picture.

YOU LIVE AS YOU EAT
People with Type A blood have digestive tracts which find it difficult to break down animal fats and proteins. Type As and Type ABs should adhere to a diet high in fibre and low in animal products.

There are specific foods which must be given extra consideration as cancer preventives.

Soya beans
Five per cent of every cake of tofu is composed of soya-bean agglutinins. Soya bean agglutinins are able to selectively identify early mutated cells producing the Type A antigen and sweep them from the system – while leaving normal Type A cells alone.

The soya bean agglutinin especially discriminates when it comes to breast cancer cells; it is so specific that it's been used to remove cancerous cells from harvested bone marrow. In experimental work with breast cancer patients, their bone marrow was removed. They were then bombarded with high levels of chemotherapy and radiation. These oncology tools would normally destroy the bone marrow. Instead, the harvested marrow – cleansed by the soya bean lectin – was then reintroduced into the patients.

These treatments have shown some very good results. The soya bean lectin also contains the oestrogen-related compounds genestein and diziden. These compounds not only help to balance the effect of a woman's oestrogen levels, but also contain other properties which can help reduce the blood supply to tumour cells.

Soya beans in all forms are beneficial to Type As and Type ABs as a general cancer preventative. The vegetable proteins in soya are easier for these blood types to utilize, and so it is strongly suggested that these blood types re-examine any aversion they may have to tofu and tofu products. Think of tofu not only as a food, but as a powerful medicine. Although Type Bs can eat soya foods, it is not certain whether they have the same action in the Type B bloodsteam.

Japanese women have such a low incidence of breast cancer because the use of tofu and other soya products is still high in the overall Japanese diet. As the diet becomes more Westernized, it is possible that we will see a proportionate rise in certain forms of cancer. One study of Japanese immigrant women living in San Francisco showed that they had twice the rate of breast cancer as their cousins living in Japan – no doubt due to change in dietary habits.

Peanuts

The peanut agglutinin has also been found to contain a specific lectin to breast cancer cells, particularly the medullary form. The peanut lectin shows activity to a lesser degree against all other forms, including intraductal lobular, and scirrhous breast cancers. This connection is probably true of other A-like cancers.

Eat fresh peanuts with the skins still on them (the skins, not the shells). Peanut butter is probably not a good source of the lectin, as the majority of brands are just too processed and homogenized.

Lentils

The *Lens culinaris* lectin found in common domestic brown or green lentils shows a strong specific attraction to lobular, medullary, intraductal, and stromal forms of breast cancer, and is likely to affect other A-like cancers.

Lima beans

Lima bean lectin is one of the most potent agglutinants of all Type A cells, cancerous or not. When you're healthy, lima beans will have a damaging effect so they shouldn't be part of a prevention strategy. However, if you are suffering from an A-like cancer, eat the lima beans. The lectin will agglutinate untold numbers of cancer cells. It will also destroy some perfectly innocent and upstanding Type A cells, but the exchange is worth it.

Wheatgerm

Wheatgerm agglutinin shows a great affinity for Type A cancers. The wheatgerm agglutinin is concentrated in the seed coating, the outer husk that is usually discarded. Unprocessed wheat bran will provide the most significant quantity of the lectin, although you can also use commercial wheatgerm preparations.

Snails

If you're Type A or Type AB, order *escargots* the next time you dine at a French restaurant. Consider it medicine packaged in a glamorous, delicious form.

The edible snail *Helix pomatia* is a powerful breast cancer agglutinin capable of determining whether the cancerous cells will metastasize (spread) to the lymph nodes.

Unless the thought of eating snails disgusts you (and really, they're quite delicious), what harm can it do?

OTHER STRATEGIES

Take care of your liver and colon

Women should be aware that the liver and colon are two major sites where oestrogens can be degraded – if their functions are disturbed the levels of oestrogen throughout the body can rise. Elevated oestrogen activity can stimulate growth of cancerous cells.

Adopt a high fibre diet to increase the levels of butyrate in the colon wall cells. Butyrates, as you may recall, promote the normalization of tissue.

The grain amaranth also contains a lectin which has a specific affinity to colon cancer cells and will destroy them.

The pneumococcus vaccine

The pneumococcus vaccine elevates anti-Type A antibodies. Type Os and Type Bs produce higher levels of anti-A antibodies when given this vaccine, which may make them better able to fight A-like cancers. In effect, it can strengthen your defences against A-like cancerous mutations, which may mean you are better prepared to fight specific cancers like breast, stomach, liver, and pancreatic cancers.

Type As will obviously not produce anti-A antibodies, but the pneumococcus vaccine may give a boost to their immune systems, helping them to recognize cancerous cells normally incognito. Since most cancers have A-like tendencies, this vaccine may, by elevating anti-Type A antibodies, mobilize the immune systems of all the blood types.

This vaccine can generate isohemmaglutinis which are much more powerful antibodies than those the body manufactures against a virus or a bacteria. Isohemmaglutinins are 'Terminators'. They agglutinate and kill their prey unaided, requiring no assistance from the other normal killer cells of the immune system.

Blood Type O and Type B may be able to increase their anti-A antibodies with a pneumococcus vaccine every 8–10 years. Blood Type A and Type AB should revaccinate more often – every 5 years.

Antioxidants

There has been so much conflicting information about antioxidants, their alleged benefits or lack of them, that it's difficult to recommend the best combinations.

Vitamin antioxidants have been studied for breast cancer, and have been shown to be not very effective in preventing the disease. Vitamin E and beta-carotenes don't deposit high enough concentrations in breast tissue to effect positive change.

The plant-based antioxidants do seem to make some difference, but must be combined with supplemental sources of vitamin C to synergize for greatest effect. Yellow onions contain very high levels of quercetin, an especially potent antioxidant. It has none of the oestrogenizing activity of vitamin E, and is hundreds of times stronger than vitamin antioxidants. Quercetin is available as a supplement in many health food shops.

Women with a risk factor for breast cancer who are considering, or are on oestrogen replacement therapy, should use phyto-oestrogens derived from natural products instead of synthetic oestrogens. Plant-based oestrogens contain high levels of oestriol, a weaker form of the oestrogen hormone than oestradiol, which is manufactured synthetically. Oestriol seems to lower your chances of developing breast cancer, whereas the synthetics increase the risk.

Tamoxifen, an oestrogen-blocking drug prescribed to breast cancer patients with oestrogen-sensitive breast tumours, is itself a weaker form of oestrogen. Genestein is an oestrogen-related compound found in the soya bean lectin. The phyto-oestrogen inhibits angiogenesis, interfering with the production of new blood vessels needed to feed the growth of cancerous tumours.

General advice
Exercise frequently, and get adequate rest. Avoid known pollutants and pesticides. Eat plenty of fruit and vegetables. Type As and Type ABs should eat plenty of tofu. Don't use antibiotics indiscriminately. If you get sick, allow your immune system to fight off the illness. You'll be much healthier if you do, rather than relying on flu or antibiotics. They suppress your immune system's potential for powerful natural responses.

* * *

Case History: Advanced breast cancer
Jane, 50: Type AB

I first saw Jane in my office in April 1993. She had already had a mastectomy and several rounds of chemotherapy for an infiltrating ductal breast cancer which had extensively seeded into the lymph nodes. At the time of her initial diagnosis, Jane had two separate tumours on her left breast – one 4 cm and the other 1.5 cm. No one was holding out any great hope for her long-term survival.

I put Jane on the modified cancer diet for Type AB, with an emphasis on soya, (high in A lectins), had her Pneumovaxed and put her on the botanical protocol I use for Type As with breast cancer. Her tumour marker, the CA15-3, which was 166 when she came in (normal is less than 10), dropped almost immediately to 87 in June, to 34 in August. I recommended that she go and see George Springer in Chicago to see if she could get into his vaccine study, which she did.

To this day all signs, including bone scans, look promising, although as a Type AB, I would be wary to pronounce Jane cured at this point. Only time will tell.

* * *

Cancer prevention and natural immune system enhancement offer the brightest hope for the future. Genetic research is bringing us ever closer to being able to understand – perhaps one day even control – the cellular workings of this astounding machine that we call our body.

Scientists at the National Institute of Allergy and Infectious Disease in Bethesda, Maryland, USA, announced on 9 May 1996, that they had found a protein used to allow the AIDS virus entry into the immune system. This discovery could be used one day to test new drugs and vaccines targeted at the AIDS virus and many cancers. This exciting breakthrough also helps to explain why some people infected with the AIDS virus remain healthy and disease-free for years, while others quickly succumb to its ravages. Wouldn't it be remarkable if the tragic scourge of AIDS led us to a cure for cancer?

Cancer has long been among the most dreaded diseases of mankind. We seem powerless to protect ourselves and those we love from its clinging and relentless grip. Blood type analysis allows us a deeper understanding of our susceptibilities. By consciously examining our exposure to both environmental and dietary carcinogens, and by changing some of our lifestyle and food choices, we can minimize the effects of cell damage.

Blood type analysis also provides a way to enhance the ability of the immune system to search out and destroy cancerous and mutated cells while they are few in number. Cancer patients can use their knowledge of blood type to fully develop the capabilities of their immune system to fight the disease. They can also gain a greater understanding of the mechanisms involved in the growth and spread of cancer.

The treatments for cancer are still far from perfect, although many people have been saved by the latest advances in therapy and scientific medical knowledge. For those of you with cancer, and for those of you who have a family history of cancer, the advice is clear: change your diet, change your attitudes, and start using antioxidant supplements. If you follow these suggestions you will be able to gain more control and a greater peace of mind. We all dread this horrible disease, but we can take positive action against it.

Epilogue
A Wrinkle of Earth

THE HUMAN JOURNEY began as one people of one blood–Type O, the blood of our first ancestors. It is an ineffable mystery as to precisely when the first Type A appeared, or the mother and father of Type B, or even when the very recent Type AB was first created. We just don't know; we can only see the broad brushstrokes of history, not its fine details.

But we are always learning. Today, the Human Genome Project employs the most sophisticated technologies in its quest to map the entire genetic structure of the human body – to name, gene by gene, chromosome by chromosome, the purpose of each living cell in the grand scheme of some Master Builder. Thus far, many breakthroughs have come in our understanding of the vast cellular networks of which we are composed – among them, the discovery of a gene for breast cancer. In late May of 1996 the Project announced that they had just isolated and identified the gene responsible for arthritis. Soon, we will be able to control our genetic fates as never before.

Or will we?

Evolution can be defined as an unfolding over time. In the waning days of the twentieth century, what is there left for us to unfold? The Hubble Telescope peers into the farthest reaches of a seemingly endless universe aswhirl in uncharted galaxies; scientists then announce that 400 or 500 billion more galaxies exist than they had previously calculated. They also announce that the observable universe extends at least 15 billion light-years – in every direction.

The Worldwide Web beckons. Communications have become

almost instantaneous. There has been an explosion of knowledge in all fields, with much more to come. We are a sophisticated, increasingly urbane people. We are at our genetic peak!

Well, so were the Neanderthals once. And for many thousands of years, Cro-Magnon dominated this planet. When the barbarian hordes came rampaging through Europe in wave after wave of invasion, it must have seemed to those invaded as if it would never end. But our lives and our memories are short. We are without substance in the flame of endless time, gossamer shredding in the wind. The revolution is not over. It is still taking place.

Evolution is very subtle. Our genetic makeups and those of our children, and those of our children's children, continue to alter in infinitesimal and unknown ways of which we are completely unaware. Some may believe that the evolution revolution is over. I am convinced that it is an ongoing, kinetic process.

The Revolution Continues

Where does the power of life come from? What propels us and compels us to survive?

Our blood. Our life force.

There have been recent outbreaks of rare viruses and infectious diseases as we have pushed into the remaining untouched jungles of this planet. These diseases defy medical intervention. Will our bodies produce answers to the challenges posed by the unknown?

This is what we face:

- Increasing ultraviolet radiation caused by the depletion of the ozone layer
- The increased pollution of our air and water
- Increasing food contamination
- Overpopulation and famine
- Infectious diseases beyond our power to control
- Unknown plagues emerging from all of the above

We will survive. We have always survived. What form that

survival will take, and what the world and its stresses will be like for the survivors, we do not know.

Perhaps a new blood type will emerge – call it Type C. This new blood type will be able to create antibodies to fend off every antigen that exists today, and any future permutation of antigens that develops. In an overcrowded, polluted world with few natural resources left, the new Type Cs will come to dominate their societies. The antiquated blood types will begin to die off in an increasingly hostile environment for which they are no longer suited. Finally, Type C will rule.

Or maybe a different scenario will be played out, one in which our scientific knowledge finally allows us to gain dominion over the worst impulses of humanity, and civilization is able to rouse itself from the suicidal impulses that seem to impel it to doom.

Our knowledge is truly vast, and there is every reason to hope that the finest and most altruistic minds and spirits of our age might focus on a way to deal with the realities of our world – violence, war, crime, ignorance, intolerance, hatred, and disease – and thus pull us out of this toxic spiral.

Nothing is complete. This world and our purpose in it is an ever-changing equation of which each of us is momentarily an integral part. The revolution continues with us or without us. Time sees us only as a blink of the eye, and it is this impermanence that makes our lives so precious.

By sharing my father's fascination with and my scientific knowledge of the Blood Type diets, I hope to make a positive impact on the life of everyone who examines this book.

Like my father before me, I am a practising naturopathic doctor. I have dedicated myself to the pursuit of naturopathic knowledge and research, and this work has been my passion for many years. It began as a gift from my father and became, for me, a gift to my father. This is the Blood Type Plan, the revolutionary breakthrough that will change the way you eat and live.

Afterword
A Medical Breakthrough for the Ages

by Dr Joseph Pizzorno, President, Bastyr University

THIS IS AN incredibly exciting time for natural medicine. Finally, modern medical science has developed the analytical tools and information base to understand the mechanisms of centuries-old healing wisdom. While many theories on health prevail worldwide, only a small number have been subjected to scientific scrutiny, as few natural healers have either the technical skills or the emotional inclination to study the research literature. For natural medicine to become established as an integral part of today's healthcare systems, it must fulfil the expectations of the modern world for reliability and credibility.

Bastyr University in Seattle, Washington, USA, has shown how to do this. Founded in 1978, Bastyr's mission has been to bring to the world the benefits of credible, science-based natural medicine. Bastyr provides accredited cutting-edge education, insightful research and effective clinical services in naturopathic medicine. Its graduates are leaders in their fields.

Dr Peter D'Adamo, a graduate of our first class of naturopathic doctors in 1982, is an outstanding example of the best Bastyr has to offer. His exciting pioneering work could change the practice of medicine for centuries to come. Inspired by his father's preliminary theories about the importance of blood type in predicting a person's biochemistry, Peter worked with students at Bastyr for over a decade culling over 1,000 papers from the scientific research literature. This exhaustive study of the medical and anthropological research, combined with clinical observation and scientific inquiry, matured into a cohesive theory with a credible foundation. The rational guidelines Peter developed will fundamentally enhance people's health and afford a deeper understanding of how an individual's genetic background determines his biochemistry and dictates his susceptibility to disease and environmental factors, including diet. This work will surely provide valuable insights for doctors responsible for the treatment of many of today's most challenging diseases.

I was first exposed to the unique concept of using blood types to better understand an individual's unique dietary and biochemical needs when Peter was a student at Bastyr. One of the courses I taught in the naturopathic medicine programme required students to carefully research a topic of interest to them and then present it, in both written and oral form, to the rest of the class. During a particularly memorable class in 1981, Peter stimulated considerable excitement and intense discussion when he presented the unexpected concept his father had intuitively developed – that blood type could be a determining factor in health. As might be expected, many more questions were asked than Peter could answer. The high level of interest and large number of insightful questions appeared to especially engage Peter's own intellectual curiosity, stimulating him to commence his important quest.

Over the next few years, Peter engaged in a considerable amount of study and research. I remember many fascinating conversations with him resulting in my recruiting several of our better graduate students at Bastyr to help him comb the medical and anthropological research journals. As the years progressed, Peter called often to share his excitement as he uncovered the surprising amount of relevant research that had been performed in a wide range of disciplines. But until Peter, no one had put it all together or thought through the implications of what different researchers were discovering.

His studies culminated in his landmark presentation at the 1989 Annual Convention of the American Association of Naturopathic Physicians in Rippling River, Oregon. The audience was extremely excited by the clinical applicability and a lively discussion followed. Since then many leading clinicians have adopted Peter's blood type-based protocols.

Hippocrates is said to have stated: 'Let your medicines be your foods and your foods your medicine.' But how to do this? One of the most significant challenges facing the dedicated physician is how to determine the best diet to recommend to his or her patients. While it is relatively easy to tell everyone to eat a balanced diet of organically grown whole foods in as natural a form as possible, this ignores the biochemical uniqueness of each individual. Genetic and environmental factors dramatically alter a person's metabolism and without ways of objectively assessing these changes, all a physician can do is guess or blindly apply the latest theory. Over the centuries, many theories about how to optimize one's diet have come and gone, but none have survived the test of time, for none have been based on scientific research. Thanks to the pioneering work of Dr Peter D'Adamo, and his father, Dr James D'Adamo, this has now changed. Here is testimony to the fact that original ideas combined with a rigorous scientific perspective can change the course of medicine.

Joseph Pizzorno, N.D.
Seattle, Washington
June 1996

Dr Pizzorno, President of Bastyr University in Seattle, Washington, the first accredited, multidisciplinary college of natural medicine in the United States, is a leading figure in the field of natural medicine. As senior editor and co-author of the internationally acclaimed A Textbook of Natural Medicine, *and the bestseller,* Encyclopedia of Natural Medicine, *he helped define the standard of care for naturopathic medicine, documented the scientific validity of natural medicine, and pushed forward the frontiers of natural healing.*

In 1993, Dr Pizzorno was invited to make a presentation on the role of naturopathic medicine in healthcare to First Lady Hillary Clinton's Health Care Reform Task Force. He was appointed to the US Congress's Office of Technology Assessments Advisory Panel on the safety and efficacy of dietary supplements, and became a consultant to the US Federal Trade Commission.

Appendix A
Blood Type Charts

TYPE O
The Hunter

strong
self-reliant
leader

Strengths	Weaknesses	Medical Risks	Diet Profile	Weight Loss Key	Supplements	Exercise
Hardy digestive tract •	Intolerant to new dietary, environmental conditions •	Blood clotting disorders •	High protein: Meat eaters •	*AVOID:* wheat corn kidney beans navy beans lentils cabbage Brussels sprouts cauliflower mustard greens	vitamin B vitamin K calcium iodine liquorice kelp	Intense physical exercise, such as: *aerobics *martial arts *contact sports *running
Strong immune system •	Immune system can be OVER active and attack itself •	Inflammatory diseases – arthritis	meat fish vegetables fruit			
Natural defences against infections •		Low thyroid production •	Limited: grains beans legumes	*AIDS:* kelp seafood salt liver red meat kale spinach broccoli		
System designed for efficient metabolism and preservation of nutrients		Ulcers • Allergies •				

TYPE A
The Cultivator

settled
co-operative
orderly

Strengths	Weaknesses	Medical Risks	Diet Profile	Weight Loss Key	Supplements	Exercise
Adapts well to dietary and environmental changes •	Sensitive digestive tract •	Heart disease •	Vegetarian •	*AVOID:* meat dairy products kidney beans lima beans wheat •	vitamin B12	Calming, centring exercises, such as:
Immune system preserves and metabolizes nutrients more easily •	Vulnerable immune system, open to microbial invasion	Cancer •	vegetables tofu seafood grains beans pulses fruit	*AIDS:* vegetable oil soya foods vegetables pineapple	folic acid	*yoga
		Anaemia •			vitamin C	*t'ai chi
		Type I diabetes			vitamin E	
					hawthorn	
					echinacea	
					quercetin	
					milk thistle	

TYPE B
The Nomad

balanced
flexible
creative

Strengths	Weaknesses	Medical Risks	Diet Profile	Weight Loss Key	Supplements	Exercise
Strong immune system •	No natural weaknesses, but imbalance causes tendency towards autoimmune breakdowns and rare viruses	Type I diabetes •	Balanced omnivore •	*AVOID:* corn lentils peanuts sesame seeds buckwheat wheat •	magnesium liquorice gingko lecithin	Moderate physical, with mental balance – such as: *hiking *cycling *tennis *swimming
Versatile adaptation to dietary and environmental changes •		Chronic Fatigue Syndrome (ME) •	meat (no chicken) dairy products grains beans pulses vegetables fruit	*AIDS:* greens eggs venison liver tea liquorice		
Balanced nervous system		Autoimmune disorders – Lou Gehrig's disease, lupus, multiple sclerosis				

TYPE AB
The Enigma

rare
charismatic
mysterious

Strengths	Weaknesses	Medical Risks	Diet Profile	Weight Loss Key	Supplements	Exercise
Designed for modern conditions •	Sensitive digestive tract •	Heart disease •	Mixed diet in moderation •	*AVOID:* red meat kidney beans lima beans seeds corn buckwheat •	vitamin C hawthorn echinacea valerian quercetin milk thistle	Calming, centring exercises, such as: *yoga *t'ai chi
Highly tolerant immune system •	Tendency for overtolerant immune system – allowing microbial invasion •	Cancer •	meat seafood dairy products tofu beans pulses grains vegetables fruit	*AIDS:* tofu seafood dairy products greens kelp pineapple		Combined with moderate physical, such as: *hiking *cycling *tennis
Combines benefits of Type A and Type B •	Reacts negatively to A-like and B-like conditions	Anaemia				

Appendix B
Common Questions

IT HAS BEEN my experience that most people respond with great enthusiasm and curiosity when they learn about the blood type connection. Yet it is far easier to embrace a provocative idea than it is to immerse oneself in the gritty details.

The Blood Type Plan is revolutionary, and as such requires many fundamental adjustments. Some people find it easier than others, depending on how much they're already living according to the needs of their blood type. Most of the questions people ask me have similar themes. I've included the most common ones here. They may help you get a clearer sense of what this diet will mean for you.

Where does my blood type come from?

Blood is universal, yet it is also unique. Like the colour of your eyes or hair, your blood type is determined by two sets of genes – the inheritance you receive from your mother and father. It is from those genes commingling that your blood type is selected, at the moment of your conception.

Like genes, some blood types are dominant over others. In the cellular creation of a new human being, Type A and Type B are dominant over Type O. If at conception the embryo is given an A gene from the mother and an O gene from the father, the infant will be Type A, although it will continue to carry the father's O gene unexpressed in its DNA. When the infant grows up and passes these genes to its offspring, half of the genes will be for Type A blood and half will be for Type O blood.

Because A and B genes are equally strong, you are Type AB if you received an A gene from one parent and a B gene from the other. Finally, because the O gene is recessive to all the others, you are Type O only if you receive an O gene from each parent.

It is possible for two Type A parents to conceive a child who is Type O. This happens when the parents each have one A gene and one O gene and both pass the O gene on to the offspring. In the same way two brown-eyed parents can conceive a blue-eyed offspring if each carries the sleeping recessive gene for blue eyes.

Blood type genetics can sometimes be used to help determine the paternity of a child. There is one catch, however. Blood type can only prove that a man is not the father of a child. It cannot be used to prove that a man *is* the child's father (although newer DNA technology can do that). Consider this example, a paternity case: An infant is Type A, the mother is Type O, and the man alleged to be the father is Type B. As both A and B genes are dominant to O, the child's father could not be Type B. Think about it. The child's A gene could not have come from the father, who, because he was Type B, would have either two B genes or a B gene and an O gene. Nor could the A gene come from the mother, because people with Type O blood always carry two O genes. The A gene had to come from someone else. These were the exact circumstances surrounding the famous paternity suit against Charlie Chaplin in 1944. Unfortunately, Chaplin was subjected to a tumultuous trial, because the use of blood type to determine paternity was not yet acceptable in a California court of law. Even though blood type had clearly shown that Chaplin was not the father of the child, the jury still decided in favour of the mother, and he was forced to pay child support.

How do I find out my blood type?

To find out your blood type, you can donate blood, or you can call your doctor to see if your blood type is in your medical file. If you'd like to test your own blood type, you can do so by ordering a finger-stick test from the following address:

Peter D'Adamo, N.D.

P.O. Box 2106

Norwalk, CT 06852–2106

Do I have to make all of the changes at once for my Blood Type Diet to work?

No. On the contrary, I suggest you start slowly, gradually eliminating the foods that are not good for you, and increasing those that are highly beneficial. Many diet programmes urge you to plunge in headfirst and radically change your lifestyle immediately. I think it's more realistic and ultimately more effective if you engage in a learning process. Don't just take my word for it. You have to learn it in your body.

Before you begin your Blood Type Diet, you may know very little about which foods are good or bad for you. You're used to making your choices according to your taste buds, family traditions, and fad diet books. Chances are you are eating some foods that are good for you, but the Blood Type Diet provides you with a powerful tool for making informed choices every time.

Once you know what your optimal eating plan is, you have the freedom to veer from your diet on occasion. Rigidity is the enemy of joy; I certainly am not a proponent of it. The Blood Type Diet is designed to make you feel great, not miserable and deprived. Obviously, there are going to be times when common sense tells you to relax the rules a bit – like when you're eating at a relative's house.

I'm Blood Type A and my husband is Blood Type O. How do we cook and eat together? I don't want to prepare two separate meals.

My wife, Martha, and I have exactly the same situation. Martha is Type O and I am Type A. We find that we can usually share about two-thirds of a meal. The main difference is in the protein source. For example, if we make a stir-fry, Martha might separately prepare some chicken, while I'll add cooked tofu. We have also found that many Type O and Type A foods are beneficial for both of us, so we emphasize those foods. For example, we might have a meal that includes salmon, rice, and broccoli. It has become relatively easy for us because we are quite familiar with the specifics of each other's Blood Type Diet. It will help you to spend some time getting familiar with your spouse's food lists. You can even make a separate list of foods that you can share. You might be surprised at how many there are.

People worry a lot about what they fear will be impossible limitations on the Blood Type Diet. But think about it. There are more than two hundred foods listed for each diet – many of them compatible across the board. Considering that the average person eats only about twenty-five foods, the Blood Type Diets actually offer more, not fewer, options.

My family is Italian, and you know the kinds of foods we like to eat. Being Type A, I don't see how I can still enjoy my favourite Italian foods – especially, no tomato sauce!

We tend to associate ethnic foods with one or two of the most commonly available – like spaghetti with meat balls and tomato sauce. But the Italian diet, like most others, includes a wide variety of different foods. Many southern Italian dishes, usually prepared with olive oil instead of heavy sauces, are wonderful choices for both Type A and Type AB. Instead of a plate of pasta drenched in red sauce, try the more delicate flavours of olive oil and garlic, a complex pesto, or a light white wine sauce. Fresh fruits or flavourful but light Italian ices are preferable to rich pastries.

My seventy-year-old husband has a history of heart problems, and has had bypass surgery. He still has a hard time staying away from the wrong foods. He's Type B and I think the Type B Diet would be perfect for him. But he's very resistant to Diets. Is there a good way to introduce the diet without a lot of fuss?

It isn't easy to radically change your diet at age seventy – which is probably why your husband has had so much trouble eating healthily, even after surgery. Rather than nagging, which is usually counterproductive, begin to gradually incorporate the beneficial Type B foods into his diet, while slowly eliminating those that aren't good for Type Bs. It's likely that your husband will develop preferences for the good foods as his digestive tract adjusts to their positive qualities.

Why do you list different portion recommendations according to ancestry?

The portion listings according to ancestry are merely refinements to the diet that you may find helpful. In the same way that men, women, and children have different portion standards, so too do people according to their body size and weight, geography, and cultural food preferences. These suggestions will help you until you are comfortable enough with the diet to naturally eat the appropriate portions.

The portion recommendations also take into account specific problems that people of different ancestries tend to have with food. African-Americans, for example, are often lactose intolerant, and most Asians are unaccustomed to eating dairy foods, so they may have to introduce these foods slowly to avoid negative reactions.

I'm allergic to peanuts, but you say they're a highly beneficial food for my blood type. Are you saying I should eat them? I'm Type A.

No. Type As have plenty of great protein sources without peanuts. These reactions are generated by the immune system, which creates antibodies that resist the food. Chances are, a person with Type A blood would not be allergic to peanuts, which contain friendly, A-like properties. You may, however, be intolerant to peanuts. That means you have digestive distress when you eat them. This could be caused by any number of factors, including an overall poor diet. Maybe you once ate peanuts, along with other problem foods, and blamed the peanuts.

Again, you don't need to include peanuts in your diet, but you may find that you tolerate them quite well once you've adjusted to the Type A Diet.

I'm Type B and my meat choices are very strange to me. It looks as though all I can eat are lamb, mutton, venison, and rabbit – which I NEVER eat. Why no chicken?

The elimination of chicken is the toughest adjustment for most people I've treated who are Type B. Not only is chicken a protein staple of many ethnic groups, but most of us have been conditioned to think that chicken is healthier than beef and other meats. Once again, however, there is no single rule that works for everyone. Chicken contains a lectin in its muscle meat that is very detrimental to Type Bs. On the brigher side, you can eat turkey and a wide variety of seafood.

What does 'neutral' mean? Are these foods good for me?

The three categories are designed to focus on the foods which are most and least beneficial to you, according to your blood type reaction to certain lectins. The highly beneficial foods act as a medicine; the foods to avoid act as a poison. The neutral foods simply act as foods. While the neutral foods may not have the special health benefits of some other foods, they're certainly good for you in the sense that they contain many nutrients that your body needs.

Must I eat all of the foods marked 'highly beneficial'?

It would be impossible to eat everything on your diet! Think of your Blood Type Diet as a painter's palette from which you may choose colours in different shades and combinations. However, do try to reach the weekly amount of the various food groups if possible. Frequency is probably more important than the individual portion sizes, so if you are Type O and have a very small build, try to have animal protein five to seven times weekly, but cut back on the portions, perhaps using two to three ounces instead of four to five ounces. This ensures that the most valuable nutrients will continue to be delivered into the bloodstream at a constant rate.

Is food combining helpful on the Blood Type Diet?

Some diet plans recommend food combining, which involves eating certain food groups in combination for better digestion. Many of these books are full of bunk and hokum, with a lot of unnecessary rules and regulations. Perhaps the only real food-combining rule is to avoid eating animal proteins, such as meats, with large amounts of starches, such as breads and potatoes. This is important because animal products are digested in the stomach in a high-acid environment, while starches are digested in the intestines in a high-alkaline environment. When these foods are combined, the body alternately nibbles at the protein, then the starch, then back to the protein, then back to the starch; not a very efficient method. By keeping these food groups separated, the stomach can concentrate its full functions on the job at hand. Substitute low-starch, high-fibre vegetable side dishes, such as greens. Protein-starch avoidance doesn't apply to tofu and other vegetable proteins, which are essentially predigested.

What should I do if a 'food to avoid' is the fourth or fifth ingredient in a recipe?

That depends on the severity of your condition, or the degree of your commpliance. If you have food allergies, or colitis, you may want to practise complete avoidance. Many high-compliance patients avoid these foods altogether, although I think this might be too extreme. Unles they suffer from a specific allergic condition, it won't hurt most people to occasionally eat a food that is not on their diet.

Will I lose weight on the Blood Type Diet?

When you read your Blood Type Plan, you will find specific recommendations for weight loss. They differ from blood type to blood type. That's because the lectins in various foods have a different effect. For example, for Type O, meat is efficiently digested and metabolized, while for Type A it slows the digestive and metabolic processes.

Your Blood Type Diet is tailor made to eliminate any imbalances that lead to weight gain. If you follow your Blood Type Diet, your metabolism will adjust to its normal level and you'll burn calories more efficiently; your digestive system will process nutrients properly and reduce water rentention. You'll lose weight immediately.

In my practice, I've found that most of my patients who have weight problems also have a history of chronic dieting. One would think that constant dieting would lead to weight loss, but that's not true if the structure of the diet and the foods it includes go against everything that makes sense for your specific body.

In our culture, we tend to promote 'one size fits all' weight-loss programmes, and then we wonder why they don't work. The answer is obvious! Different blood types respond to food in different ways. In conjunction with the recommended exercise programme, you should see results very quickly.

Do calories matter on the Blood Type Diet?

As with most general diet issues, concerns about calories are automatically taken care of by following your specific Blood Type Diet. Most new patients who follow the guidelines concerning diet and exercise lose some weight. Some people even complain that they are losing too much weight. There is an adjustment period on this diet, and over time you'll be able to find the food amounts that suit your needs. However, the charts in each food category give you a place to start.

It's important to be aware of portion sizes. No matter what you eat, if you eat too much of it you'll gain weight. This probably seems so obvious that it doesn't even bear mentioning. But overeating has become one of America's most difficult and dangerous health problems. Millions of Americans are bloated and dyspeptic because of the amounts of food they eat. When you eat excessively, the walls of your stomach stretch like an inflated balloon. Although stomach muscles are elastic and were created to contract and expand, when they are grossly enlarged the cells of the abdominal walls undergo a tremendous strain. If you are eating until you feel full, and you normally feel sluggish after a meal, try to reduce your portion sizes. Learn to listen to what your body is telling you.

I have heart problems and I've been told to totally avoid any fat and cholesterol. 'I'm Type O. How can I eat meat?

First, realize that it is grains, not meats, which are the cardiovascular culprits for Type O. This is especially interesting because almost everybody who has or is attempting to prevent heart disease is advised to go on a diet based largely on complex carbohydrates!

For Type Os, a high intake of certain carbohydrates, usually wheat breads, increases the insulin levels. In response, your body stores more fat in the tissues, and fat levels are elevated in the blood.

Also bear in mind that your blood cholesterol level is only moderately controlled by the dietary intake of foods that are high in cholesterol content. Approximately 85 to 90 per cent is actually controlled by the manufacture and metabolism of cholesterol in your liver.

I'm Type O and don't want to eat much fat in my diet. What do you suggest?

A high-protein diet does not automatically mean one that is high in fat, especially if you avoid heavily marbleized meats. Although more expensive, try to find free-range meats that have been raised without the excessive use of antibiotics and other chemicals. Our ancestors consumed rather lean game or domestic animals that grazed on alfalfa and other grasses; today's high-fat meats are produced by using high amounts of corn feed.

If you can't afford or can't find free-range meats, choose the leanest cuts available and remove all excess fat before cooking. Type Os also have many other good protein choices that are naturally lower in fat – such as chicken and seafood. The fat in the oil-rich fish is composed of omega-3 fatty acids, which seem to promote lower cholesterol and healthier hearts.

How can I be sure to buy the most natural and the freshest foods?

Within the last few years, many consumers have banded together to create food co-ops, groups of people who buy in bulk. Very often this bulk purchasing power results in great savings and high-quality produce. Most food co-ops require a small membership fee and a few hours of work at the co-op per month. Savings, especially on items such as grains, spices, beans, vegetables, and oils can be substantial.

Health food stores can be a valuable place to buy fresh foods, but don't fall into the trap of thinking that because you are in a health food store you can relax your guard. Many health food stores, especially the smaller ones, do not have the rapid turnover of a busy greengrocer or supermarket, and their foods might not be as fresh.

Are organic foods more healthy than non-organic foods?

A good rule of thumb is to use organic vegetables if they are not exorbitantly priced. They do taste better, and are more healthy. However, if you are on a fixed income and cannot find competitively priced organic produce, high-quality, properly cleaned, fresh non-organic produce will do just fine.

More and more supermarkets in America seem to be stocking organic produce, mostly from California, a state with specific laws concerning the use of the term *organic*. Interestingly, in one supermarket in my neighbourhood, organic vegetables and fruits are displayed next to the non-organic versions, and are priced identically! I suspect that market pressures will continue to push more and more vegetable and fruit growers toward the organic way, if for no other reason than the cost of commercial fertilizers, made from petro-chemicals, will eventually make them more expensive to produce than naturally grown products.

Will eating canned food hurt my diet?

Commercially canned foods, subject to high heat and pressure, lose most of their vitamin content, especially the antioxidants, such as Vitamin C. They do retain the vitamins that are not heat sensitive, such as vitamin A. Canned foods typically are lower in fibre than their fresh counterparts and higher in salt, usually added to offset the loss of flavours in production. Soggy, with little of the 'life' we find in fresh foods and vegetables, and few natsural enzymes (which are destroyed by the canning process), canned foods should be used sparingly, if at all. You pay much more per weight for canned food, and don't get back much in return.

Other than fresh, frozen foods are your best second bet. Freezing does not change the nutritional content of the food very much (its preparation before freezing may) although the taste and the texture are often blunted.

Why is stir-frying so beneficial?

The quick frying of Oriental-style cooking is healthier than deep frying. Less oil is used, and the oil itself, typically sesame oil, is more resistant to high temperatures than safflower or canola oils. The idea behind stir-frying is to quickly braise the food on its outside, which has the added effect of sealing in flavours.

Most types of meals can be prepared in this manner using a wok. The deep, cone-shaped design of the wok concentrates the heat at a small area at its base, which allows food to be cooked there and then moved to the cooler edges of the pan. Wok cooking usually mixes vegetables and seafoods or meats. Cook the meats and vegetables that require longer heating first, then move them to the outside of the pan, adding the vegetables that require less cooking to the centre.

Steaming vegetables is also a quick and effective method of cooking, and helps to keep the nutrients in the food. Use a simple steamer basket, purchased at any hardware or department store, fitted inside a large pot filled with water to the level of the basket bottom. Add vegetables, cover and heat. Don't cook until soggy! Crisp means better taste, better texture, and better nutrition.

Should I take a multivitamin every day on the Blood Type Diet?

If you are in good health and are following your Blood Type Diet, you shouldn't really need a supplement, although there are exceptions. Pregnant women should supplement their diet with iron, calcium, and folic acid. Most women also need extra calcium – especially if their diet doesn't include many dairy foods.

Those engaged in heavy physical activity, people in stressful occupations, the elderly, those who are ill, heavy smokers – all should be on a supplementation programme. More specific details are available in your individual Blood Type Plan.

How important are herbs and herbal teas?

That depends on your blood type. Type Os respond well to soothing herbs, Type As to the more stimulating ones, and Type Bs do quite nicely without most of them. Type ABs should follow the herbal protocols laid down for Type As, with the added proviso that Type ABs shun those herbs that both Type As and Type Bs are asked to avoid.

Why are vegetable oils so limited on the Blood Type Diet? I thought all vegetable oils were good for you.

What you've probably heard is advertisers hawking the news that vegetable oils have 'No Cholesterol!' Well, that's not news to anyone with even a modicum of knowledge about nutrition. Plants and vegetables do not manufacture cholesterol, which is found only in products derived from animals. Your cholesterol-free oil may have little else to recommend it.

Here are the facts. Always avoid tropical oils, such as coconut oil, as they are high in saturated fat, which can be harmful to the cardiovascular system. Most oils sold today, including safflower and canola (rapeseed) are polyunsaturated, which makes them an improvement over lard and tropical oils. However, there is some concern that overconsumption of polyunsaturated fats may be linked to certain types of cancer, especially if they're subjected to the high temperatures of cooking. In general, I prefer to use olive oil as mch as possible in cooking. I believe that olive oil has proven to be the most tolerated and beneficial of fats. As a monounsaturated oil it seems to have positive effects on the heart and arteries. There are many different blends of olive oil available. The finest quality is the extra-virgin grade. It is slightly greenish in colour and almost odourless – although when gently heated, the perfume of the olives is sensational. Olive oil is usually cold-pressed rather than extracted using heat or chemicals. The less processed an oil is, the better its quality.

Tofu seems like a very unappealing food. Must I eat it if I'm Type A?

Many Type A and Type AB people raise their eyebrows and grimace with disgust when I recommend that they make tofu a staple of their diets. Well, tofu is not a glamour food. I admit it. When I was an impoverished Type A college student, I ate tofu with vegetables and brown rice almost every day for years. It was cheap, but I actually liked it.

I think the real problem with tofu is the way it is usually displayed in the markets. Tofu – in soft or hard cakes – sits with its other tofu friends in a large plastic tub, immersed in cold water. When people manage to overcome their initial aversion and actually purchase one or two tofu cakes (calling them cakes has a rather bitter irony), many people take it home, pop it on a plate, and break off a hunk to give it a try. This is a bad way to experience tofu! It might be comparable to tossing a whole raw egg into your mouth and chewing . . . not a very pleasant experience.

If you are going to use tofu, it is best cooked and combined with vegetables and strong flavours that you enjoy, such as garlic, ginger, and soy sauce.

Tofu is a nutritionally complete meal that is filling and extremely inexpensive. Type As take note: The path to your good health is paved with bean curd!

I've never heard of many of the grains you mention. Where do I find out more?

If you're looking for alternative grains, health food stores are a bonanza. In recent years, many ancient grains, largely forgotten, have been rediscovered and are now being produced. Examples of these are amaranth, a grain from Mexico, and spelt, a variation of wheat that seems to be free of the problems found with whole wheat. Try them! They're not bad. Spelt flour makes a hearty, chewy bread that is quite flavourful, while several interesting breakfast cereals are now being made with amaranth. Another alternative is to use sprouted-wheat breads, sometimes referred to as Ezekiel or Essene bread, as the gluten lectins found principally in the seed coat are destroyed by the sprouting process. These breads spoil rapidly and are usually found in the refrigerator cases of health food stores. They are a live food, with many beneficial enzymes still intact. Beware of commercially produced sprouted wheat breads, as they usually have a minority of sprouted wheat and a majority of whole wheat in their formulas. Sprouted bread is somewhat sweet tasting, as the sprouting process also released sugars, and it is moist and chewy. This bread makes wonderful toast.

I'm type A and I've been a runner for many years. Running seems to be a great way to reduce stress. I'm confused about your advice that I shouldn'st exercise heavily.

There is a great deal of evidence that your blood type informs your unique reaction to stress, and that Type As tend to do better with less intense exercise. My father has observed this thousands of times in his thirty-five years studying the connection. However, there is much we don't yet know, so I would hesitate to say absolutely that you shouldn't run.

I would ask you to reevaluate your health and energy levels. I often have patients who say things like, 'I've always been a runner,' or 'I've always eaten chicken,' as if that were all the proof they needed that an activity or a food was beneficial. Often, these very people are suffering from an assortment of physical problems and stresses that they've never thought to associate with specific activities or foods. You may be a Type A with a twist – one who thrives on intense physical activity. Or you may discover that you're running on empty.

Appendix C
Glossary of Terms

ABO blood group system: The most important of the blood-typing systems, the ABO blood group is the determinant for transfusion reactions and organ transplantation. Unlike the other blood-typing systems, the ABO blood types have far-ranging significance other than transfusion or transplantation, including the determining of many of the digestive and immunological characteristics of the body. The ABO blood group is comprised of four blood types: O, A, B and AB. Type O has no true antigen, but carries antibodies to both A and B blood. Type A and Type B carry the antigen named for their blood type and make antibodies to each other. Type AB does not manufacture any antibodies to other blood types because it has both A and B antigens.

Anthropologists use the ABO blood types extensively as a guide to the development of early peoples. Many diseases, especially digestive disorders, cancer, and infection, express preferences, choosing between the ABO blood types. These expressions are not generally understood or appreciated by either doctors or the general population.

Agglutinate: Derived from the Latin word 'to glue'. The process by which cells are made to adhere to one another, usually through the actions of an agglutinin, such as an antibody or a lectin. Certain viruses and bacteria are also capable of agglutinating blood cells. Many agglutinins, particularly the food lectins, are blood type specific. Certain foods clump only the cells of one blood type, and do not react with the cells of another type.

Anthropology: The study of the human race in relation to distribution, origin and classification. Anthropologists study physical characteristics, the relationship of races, environmental and social relations and cultures. The ABO blood types are extensively used by anthropologists in the study of early human populations.

Antibody: A class of chemicals, called the immunoglobulins, made by the cells of the immune system to specifically tag or identify foreign material within the body of the host. Antibodies combine with specific markers – antigens – found on viruses, bacteria or other toxins, and agglutinate them. The immune system is capable of manufacturing millions of different antibodies against a wide variety of potential invaders. Individuals of Type O, Type A or Type B blood carry antibodies to other blood types. Type AB, the universal recipient, manufactures no antibodies to other types.

Antigen: Any chemical which generates an antibody by the immune system in response to it. The chemical markers which determine blood type are considered blood type antigens because other blood types may carry antibodies to them. Antigens are commonly found on the surface of germs, and are used by the immune system to detect foreign material. Specialized antigens are often made by cancer cells, these being called tumour antigens. Many germs and cancer antigens are clever impersonators which can mimic the blood type of the host in an effort to escape detection.

Antioxidant: Vitamins that are believed to strengthen the immune system and prevent cancer by fighting off toxic compounds (called free radicals) that attack cells. Vitamins C, E, and beta-carotene are believed to be the most powerful antioxidants.

Cro-Magnon: The first truly modern human. Originating around 70–40,000 BC, Cro-Magnon migrated extensively from Africa into Europe and Asia. A master hunter. Cro-Magnon led a largely hunter–gatherer existence. Most of the digestive characteristics of people with Type O blood are derived from Cro-Magnon.

Differentiation: The cellular process by which cells develop their specialized characteristics and functions. Differentiation is controlled by the genetic machinery of the cell. Cancer cells, which often have defective genes, usually de-evolve, and lose many of the characteristics of a normal cell, often reverting to earlier embryologic forms long repressed since early development.

Gene: A component of the cell which controls the transmission of hereditary characteristics by specifying the construction of a particular protein or enzyme. Genes are composed of long chains of deoxyribonucleic acid (DNA) contained in the chromosomes of the cell nucleus.

Indo-European: An early Caucasian people who migrated westward to Europe from their early homelands in Asia and the Middle East around 7000–3500 BC. The Indo-Europeans were probably the progenitors for Type A blood in western Europe.

Ketosis: A state that is achieved with a high-protein, low-carbohydrate diet. The high-protein diets of our early Type O ancestors forced the burning of fat for energy and the production of ketones – a sign of rapid metabolic activity. The state of ketosis allowed early humans to maintain high energy, metabolic efficiency, and physical strength – all qualities needed for hunting game.

Lectin: Any compound, usually a protein, found in nature, which can interact with surface antigens found on the body's cells, causing them to agglutinate. Lectins are often found in common foods, and many of them are blood type specific. Because cancer cells often manufacture copious amounts of antigens on their surface, many lectins will agglutimate them in preference to normal cells.

Mucus: Secretions manufactured by specialized tissues, called mucous membranes, which are used to lubricate and protect the delicate internal linings of the body. Mucus contains antibodies to protect against germs. In secretors, large amounts of blood type antigens are secreted in mucus, which serves to filter out bacteria, fungi and parasites with opposing blood type characteristics.

Naturopathic doctor (N.D.): A doctor trained in natural healing methods. Naturopathic doctors receive a four-year postgraduate training at an accredited college or university, and function as primary-care providers.

Neolithic: The period of early human development characterized by the development of agriculture and the use of pottery and polished tools. The radical change in human lifestyle, from the previous hunter-gatherer existence, was probably a major stimulus to the development of Blood Type A.

Panhemaglutinans: Lectins that agglutinate all blood types. An example is the tomato lectin.

Polymorphism: Literally means 'many shapes'. A polymorphism is any physical manifestation within a species of living organisms which is variable through genetic influence. The blood types are a well-known polymorphism.

Phytochemical: Any natural product with specific health applications. Most phytochemicals are traditional herbs and plants.

Triglycerides: The body's fat stores, also contained in the bloodstream. High triglycerides – or high blood fats – are considered a risk for heart disease.

Appendix D
Notes on the Anthropology
of Blood Type

ANTHROPOLOGY IS THE study of human differences, cultural and biological. Most anthropologists divide the field into two categories: cultural anthropology, which looks at the manifestations of culture, such as language or ritual; and physical anthropology, the study of the evolutionary biology of our species, *Homo sapiens*. Physical anthropologists attempt to trace human historical development through hard scientific methods, such as the blood types. A central task in physical anthropology has been to document the sequence of how the human line evolved from early primate ancestors. The use of blood types to study early societies has been termed paleoserology, the study of ancient blood.

Physical anthropology is also concerned with how humans adapted to environmental pressures. Traditional physical anthropology relied heavily on the measuring of skull shape, stature, and other physical characteristics. Blood type became a powerful tool for this type of analysis. In the 1950s, as emphasis shifted to genetic characteristics, interest shifted to the blood types and other markers that have known genetic bases. A. E. Mourant, a doctor and anthropologist, has published two key works, *Blood Groups and Disease* (Oxford Press, 1984), and *Blood Relations: Blood Groups and Anthropology* (Oxford University Press, 1983), which have collected much of the available material on the subject.

In addition to Mourant, I've used a variety of other source material for this appendix, including earlier anthropology sources such as William Boyd's *Genetics and the Races of Man* (1950), and a series of studies which were published in various journals of forensic medicine from 1920–1945.

It is possible to map the occurrence of the various blood groups in ancient populations by blood typing grave exhumations. Small amounts of blood type materials can be reconstituted from the remains, and the blood type determined. By studying the blood types of human populations, anthropologists gain information about that population's local history, movement, intermarriage, and diversification.

Many national and ethnic groups have unique blood type distributions. In certain more isolated cultures, a clear majority of one blood type over another can still be seen. In other societies, the distribution may be more even. In the United States, for example, the equal rates of Type O and Type A blood reflect masses of immigration. The United States also has a higher percentage of Blood Type B than the western European countries, which probably reflects the influx of more eastern nationalities.

For the purpose of this analysis, we can divide humankind into two basic races – Ethiopian and Palearctic. The Palearctic can be further broken down into Mongolians and Caucasians, although most people lie somewhere in between. Each race is physically characterized by its environment and occupies distinct geographic areas. Ethiopians, probably the oldest race, are dark-skinned Africans, inhabiting the southern third of Arabia and sub-Saharan Africa. The Palearctic region comprises Africa north of the Sahara, then Europe, most of Asia (with the exception of southern Arabia), India, South-East Asia, and southern China.

The roughest guesswork places the beginnings of human migration from Africa to Asia at about 1 million years ago. In Asia, most likely, modern *Homo sapiens* species split from a trunk of the ancestral Ethiopians into the Caucasians and Mongolians, but we know almost nothing about when or why it occurred.

Each of the basic races has its own homeland – a geographic area where it is pre-eminent. The Ethiopian homeland was Africa, the Caucasian Europe and northern Asia, and the Mongolian central and southern Asia.

As human groups migrated and interbred, intermediate populations evolved in the creases and crevices between these ancestral homelands. The area bound by the Sahara, the Middle East, and Somalia, for example, was home to a blending of the African and Caucasian races; the Indian subcontinent, a blend of the more northerly Caucasians and the more southerly Mongolians. These groups, which then split into innumerable, often temporary populations, were subject to the pressures of disease, food sources, and climate. They may have existed for thousands of years in the spaces between the homelands. Although the result of migration was to spread Type O blood far and wide around the world, it was from these spaces that the later blood types emerged.

There may be more physical differences between Africans and the other races, but the blood type differences between Caucasians and Mongolians are more clear cut – a good reason to reexamine racial stereotypes.

It would also be a mistake to think of the early Type O people as primitives. More intellectual development occurred in the Cro-Magnon age than in any time before or after. The Cro-Magnons created our early societies and rituals, more than the rudiments of communication, and the original wanderlust. Although we trace the genetic heritage of Type O blood back to early prehistory, it still remains a very workable chemistry, largely because of its simplicity and the fact that animal protein diets still account for a great portion of the world's current food intake.

The first attempt at using blood type to describe racial and nationality characteristics was undertaken by a husband-and-wife team of doctors, the Hirszfelds, in 1918. During the First World War both had served as doctors in the Allied armies that had concentrated in the area of Salonika, Greece.

Working with a multinational force, and with large amounts of refugees of different ethnic backgrounds, the Hirszfelds systematically blood typed large numbers of people while also recording their race and nationality. Each group contained over 500 or more subjects.

They found, for example, that the rate of Blood Type B ranged from a low of 7.2 per cent of the population of English subjects, to a high of 41.2 per cent in Indians, and that western

Europeans in general had a lower incidence of Type B than Balkan Slavs, who had a lower incidence than Russians, Turks and Jews; who again had a lower occurrence than Vietnamese and Indians. The distribution of Blood Type AB essentially followed the same pattern, with a low of 3–5 per cent in western Europeans, and a high of 8.5 per cent in Indians.

In subcontinental India, Type ABs make up 8.5 per cent of the population – remarkably high for a blood type that averages between 2 and 5 per cent worldwide. This prevalence of Type ABs is probably due to subcontinental India's location as an invasion route between the conquered lands to the west and the Mongolian homelands to the east.

Blood Type O and Type A were essentially the reverse of Type B and Type AB. The percentage of Type A remained fairly consistent (40 per cent) among Europeans, Balkan Slavs and Arabs, while being quite low in west Africans, Vietnamese and Indians. Forty-six per cent of the English population tested were Type O, which accounted for only 31.3 per cent of the Indians tested.

Modern analysis (largely the result of records kept by blood banks), encompasses the blood types of greater than 20 million individuals from around the world. Yet, these large numbers can do no more than confirm the original observations of the Hirszfelds. No scientific journals saw fit to publish their material at that time. For a while, the Hirszfelds' study languished in an obscure anthropology journal; for over thirty years this fascinating and important work was overlooked.

Apparently, there was little interest in using this knowledge of the blood types as an anthropological probe into the history of humanity.

RACIAL CLASSIFICATIONS BASED ON BLOOD TYPE

In the 1920s several anthropologists first attempted racial classifications based on blood groups. In 1929 Laurance Snyder published a book called *Blood Grouping In Relationship to Clinical and Legal Medicine* (Williams and Wilkin Publishers). In it, Snyder proposed a comprehensive classification system based on blood type. It is especially interesting because it largely focuses on the distribution of the ABO groups, the only tool to be had at the time.

The Racial Classifications – as Snyder saw them – were:

The European type
High frequency of Blood Type A, low frequency of Type B, perhaps the result of Type A blood originating in western Europe. This category included English, Scots, French, Belgians, Italians and Germans.

Intermediate type
A sort of blend between western (high Type A) and central (high Type B) European populations. Higher incidence of Blood Type O overall. This category included the Finns, Arabs, Russians, Spanish Jews, Armenians and Lithuanians.

Hunan type
Oriental groups with a high incidence of Blood Type A, possibly the result of an infusion of Caucasian elements, including the Ukrainians, Poles, Hungarians, Japanese, Romanian Jews, Koreans, and southern Chinese.

Indo-Manchurian type
Contains population groups with a high incidence of Blood Type B over Type A. This type includes the subcontinental Indians, Gypsies, northern Chinese, and Manchus.

Afro-Malaysian type
Moderately higher incidence of Type A and Type B overall, with normal incidence of Type O. This category includes Javanese, Sumatrans, Africans, and Moroccans.

Pacific-American type
Including Filipinos, North and South American Indians, and Eskimos. Extremely high incidence of Type O and Rh+ blood types, very small incidence of Type A, and almost absent incidence of Type B.

Australasian type

Principally the Australian Aborigines, this classification shows high incidence of Type A (almost equivalent to western Europe), almost no Type B, and a high incidence of Type O, although not as high as found in the Pacific-American type.

Because he could only rely on ABO blood types, Snyder's classifications made for some strange pairings, such as the Hunan type containing both Koreans and Romanian Jews. Later, researchers began using using the Rh and MN blood types, in addition to the ABO in their classifications, trying to refine these categories. They were aware that racial classification based merely on ABO groups would, in many cases, give results which would not coincide with older ideas about race, so they also incorporated MN types and occasional other blood factors to distinguish populations not clearly differentiated by ABO.

One classification, based on these newer criteria, distinguished the following races:

Europeans (Nordics and Alpines of Europe/Near East)
Mediterranean
Mongolian (Central Asia and Eurasia)
African
Indonesian
American Indian
Oceanic (including Japanese)
Australian

Another racial classification, based largely on ABO and Rh factors:

Caucasian group

Highest incidence of Rh−, relatively high Type A, moderately high incidence of all other blood types.

Negroid group

Highest incidence of rare Rh types, moderate frequency of Rh−, high relative incidence of Blood Type A2, and the rare intermediates of Type A–Ax and A Bantu.

Mongolian group

Virtual absence of blood types Rh− and Type A2. Using MN data further classified the Mongolian group into: Asiatic group, Pacific Island and Australian group, American Indian and Eskimo group.

William Boyd, in his 1950 book *Genetics And The Races of Man* (Little, Brown and Co.), proposed a more accurate system based on this earlier classification:

Early European group

Possessing the highest incidence (over 30 per cent) of the Rh−, and probably no Type B. A relatively high incidence of Blood Type O. The gene for subtype N possibly somewhat higher than in present-day Europeans. Represented today by their modern descendants, the Basques.

European (Caucasoid) group

Possessing the next highest incidence of the Rh− and a relatively high incidence of Blood Type A2, with moderate frequencies of other blood group genes. Normal frequencies of the gene for subtype M.

African (Negroid) group

Possessing a tremendously high incidence of a rare Rh+ blood type gene, Rh0, and a moderate frequency of Rh−; relatively high incidence of Type A2 and the rare intermediate Types of A, and a rather high incidence of Blood Type B.

Asiatic (Mongolian) group

Possessing high frequencies of Blood Type B, but little if any of the genes for Blood Type A2 and Rh−.

American Indian group

Possessing little or no Type A, and probably no Type B or Rh−. Very high rates of Blood Type O.

Australoid group
Possessing high incidence of Blood Type A1, but not Type A2, or Rh−. High incidence of gene for N subtype.

Boyd's classification made more sense than the earlier classification systems, because it also fit the geographic distributions of the individual races more accurately.

Recent work by Dr Luigi Cavalli-Sforza at Stanford University has tracked the genetic drift of the ancient human migrations, using even more sophisticated methods based on the new DNA technology. Many of his findings have confirmed the earlier observations of Mourant, the Hirszfelds, Snyder, and Boyd concerning the distribution of blood types worldwide.

Appendix E
The Blood Type Subgroups

MORE THAN 90 PER CENT of all factors associated with blood type are related to your major ABO type. There are, however, many minor blood subtypes, most of them playing insignificant roles. Of all the subtypes, only three will have any impact on your profile or affect your health and diet. I mention them only because they occasionally pop up as a useful refinement in your health plan. But let me stress: Knowing whether you are Type O, Type A, Type B, or Type AB is the only blood type information you really need.

The three subtypes that play minor roles are:

- SECRETOR/NON-SECRETOR STATUS
- RH POSITIVE (RH+) AND RH NEGATIVE (RH)
- THE MN BLOOD GROUP SYSTEM

SECRETORS AND NON-SECRETORS

Although everyone carried a blood type antigen on their blood cells, some people also have blood type antigens tht float around freely in their body secretions. These people are called secretors, because they secrete their blood type antigens into their saliva, mucus, sperm, and other body fluids. In addition to their blood, it's possible to learn the blood type of a secretor from these other fluids. Secretors comprise about 80 per cent of the population, non-secretors 20 per cent.

Secretor status has important implications in law enforcement. A semen sample taken from a rape victim can be used to help convict the rapist if he is a secretor and his blood type matches the blood type identified in the semen. However, if he is in the small population of non-secretors, his blood type cannot be identified from any fluids except the blood.

People who do not secrete their blood type antigens in other fluids besides blood are called non-secretors. Being a secretor or a non-secretor is independent of your ABO blood type; it is controlled by a different gene. Thus one person could be a Type A secretor, and another a Type A non-secretor.

Because secretors have more places to put their blood type antigens, they have more blood type expression in their bodies than non-secretors. Finding out whether or not you are a secretor is as easy as finding out your ABO blood type. The most common way to determine secretor status involves testing saliva for the presence of blood type activity. It is not a common test, although there are several laboratories (listed in the back of the book) that will perform it for a small fee. I suggest that until you find out your secretor status for certain, play the numerical odds and assume you are a secretor.

If you are tested for secretor status, something called the Lewis System will probably be used. It's a quick-and-dirty way to identify secretors and non-secretors, and I mention it here only so you can recognize it if you see it on a blood type report.

In the Lewis System there are two possible antigens that can be produced, called Lewis a and Lewis b (not to be confused with the A and B of the ABO system), and their interplay determines your secretor status. LEWIS a+ b− equals non-secretor. LEWIS a− b+ equals secretor.

POSITIVE OR NEGATIVE

When we blood-type patients in my office, they almost immediately ask if they are negative or positive. Many people don't realize that this is an additional separate blood grouping called the Rhesus, or Rh, system, and it really has nothing to do with your ABO blood type – although it does have one important ramification for pregnant women.

The Rh system is named for rhesus monkey, a commonly used laboratory animal, in whose blood it was first discovered. For many years it remained a mystery to doctors why some women who had normal first pregnancies developed complications in their second and subsequent pregnancies, often resulting in miscarriage and even the death of the mother. In 1940, it was discovered (again by the amazing Dr Landsteiner) that these women were carrying a different blood type than their babies, who took their blood type from the father. The babies were Rh+, meaning that they carried the Rh antigen on their blood cells. Their mothers were Rh−, which meant that this antigen was missing from their blood. Unlike the ABO system, in which the antibodies to other blood types develop from birth, Rh− people do not make an antibody to the Rh antigen unless they are first sensitized. This sensitization usually occurs when blood is exchanged between the mother and infant during birth, so the mother's immune system does not have enough time to react to the first baby. However, should a subsequent conception result in another Rh+ baby, the mother, now sensitized, will produce antibodies to the baby's blood type. Reactions to the Rh factor can occur only in Rh− women who conceive the children of Rh+ fathers. Rh+ women, 85 per cent of the population, have nothing to worry about. Even though the Rh system doesn't figure prominently when it comes to diets or diseases, it is certainly a factor for childbearing women who are Rh−.

IF YOU HAVE	BUT DO NOT HAVE	YOU ARE
The Rh antigen	The anti-Rh antibody	Rh+
The anti-Rh antibody	The Rh antigen	Rh−

THE MN BLOOD GROUP SYSTEM

The MN blood group system is virtually unknown because it is not a major factor in transfusions or organ transplants, and is of little interest in the day-to-day practice of medicine. This is deceiving, however, because a variety of diseases are associated with them – if only in a minor way.

In this system, a person can type out as MM, NN, or MN, depending upon whether his or her cells have only the M antigen (which would make them MM), the N antigen (NN), or both (MN). This system will pop up occasionally in our discussions, especially when we talk about cancer and heart disease. Around 28 per cent of the population is typed as MM, 22 per cent as NN, and 50 per cent as MN.

IF YOU HAVE	BUT DO NOT HAVE	YOU ARE
The M antigen	The N antigen	Type MM
The N antigen	The M antigen	Type NN
The M and N antigens		Type MN

YOUR BLOOD TYPE PEDIGREE

These three subtype systems are often used in my office, and they are often a part of various lab panels in use by other doctors. Although you can find almost all of the information you will ever need simply by knowing your ABO type, these systems offer a further refinement that allows a much deeper understanding of your blood's characteristics.

This results in what I call the blood type pedigree, a string of letters that is a patient's profile. In many ways, it is as specific as a fingerprint. One look at the pedigree points me in the proper direction and guides me in devising a diet and disease-prevention strategies. An example of one person's pedigree is:

BLOOD TYPE	SECRETOR STATUS	NEG/POS	MN
O	Lewis a+ b− (non-secretor)	Rh−	MM

Another is:

BLOOD TYPE	SECRETOR STATUS	NEG/POS	MN
A	Lewis a– b+ (secretor)	Rh+	MN

If you wish to refine your programme to this degree, you will find laboratories and other resources in the back of this book. However, don't get sidetracked from the main point: Knowing your ABO blood type alone will give you 90 per cent of the information you need, and that should be your primary focus.

Appendix F
Resources: Getting Help

Dr. Peter D'Adamo is in private practice in Stamford, CT. For general information, to be put on a mailing list, or to comment on your own experiences with *Eat Right 4 Your Type*, please use the P.O. box number or the Internet address.

The D'Adamo Clinic, LLC
213 Danbury Road
Wilton, CT 06897
203 834 7500

Visit Dr. D'Adamo's web site for the latest blood type news at: www.dadamo.com

Peter D'Adamo's father, who pioneered much of the initial research and clinical work on blood types, is still in practice. You may reach James D'Adamo, N.D., at:

44–46 Bridge St
Portsmouth, NH 03801

For information regarding blood type specific food supplements, home test kits, educational literature and home blood-typing kits, please contact:
North American Pharmacal, Inc.
"D'Adamo Personalized Nutrition"
213 Danbury Road
Wilton, CT 06897
Tel: 203 761 0042
Fax: 203 76 0043
Toll-Free: 1 877-ABO-TYPE (1 877 226 8973)
www.4yourtype.com

Physicians wishing to apply the blood-typing system in the USA can order testing from:
Dr. Thomas Kruzel, ND, MT.
800 SE 181st Ave
Gresham, OR 97233
(503) 667 1961

The official UK distributor of Dr D'Adamo's Home Blood Type Kits and Blood Type Speciality Products is:
Stacktheme Ltd
59 Bridge Street
Dollar
Scotland
FK14 7DQ

TEL: 01259 743255
FAX: 01259 743002
EMAIL: info@stacktheme.com

Appendix G
References

RATHER THAN FILL this book with endless footnotes, I've collected the most important influences on it and listed them here where they might be most easily referred to. They are grouped into several categories and listed alphabetically by author.

Blood types, general information

American Association of Blood Banks. *Technical Manual*, 10th ed. 1990.

D'Adamo, P. 'Gut ecosystems III: The ABO and other polymorphic systems.' *Townsend Ltr. for Doctors*, Aug. 1990.

Marcus, D. M. 'The ABO and Lewis blood-group system.' *New England J. Med.*, 280 (1969): 994–1005.

Diet and lifestyle

Atkins, R., and Herwood, R. W. *Dr Atkins's Diet Revolution*. New York: Bantam, 1972.

D'Adamo, J. *The D'Adamo Diet*. Montreal: McGraw-Hill Ryerson, 1989.

——. *One Man's Food*. New York: Marek, 1980. (out of print).

Kushi, M., and Jack, A. *The Cancer Prevention Diet*. New York: St Martin's, 1983.

Nomi, T., and Besher, A. *You Are Your Blood Type*. New York: Pocket, 1983.

Pritikin, N., and McGrady, P. *The Pritikin Program for Diet and Exercise*. New York: Grosset & Dunlap, 1979.

Schmid, R., *Traditional Foods Are Your Best Medicine*. New York: Balantine, 1987.

Blood types and anthropology

Boyd, W. C. *Genetics and the Races of Man: An Introduction to Modern Physical Anthropology.* Boston: Little, Brown, 1950.

Brues, A. M., 'Tests of blood group selection.' *Amer. J. Forensic Medicine*, 1929: 287–89.

Childe, V. G. *Man Makes Himself.* London: Watts, 1936.

Coon, C. S. *The Races of Europe.* New York: Macmillan, 1939.

Gates, R. R. *Human Ancestry.* Cambridge, MA: Harvard University Press, 1948.

Hirszfeld, L., and Hirszfeld, H. *Lancet*, 2 (1919): 675.

Livingstone, F. R. 'Natural selection disease and ongoing human evolution as illustrated by the ABO groups.' Source unknown (copy in author's possession).

McNeil, W. H. *Plagues and Peoples.* New York: Doubleday/Anchor, 1975.

Mourant, A. E. *Blood Relations: Blood Groups and Anthropology.* Oxford, England: Oxford University Press, 1983.

——, Kopec, A. C., and Domaniewska-Sobczak, K. *Blood Groups and Disease*, Oxford England: Oxford University Press, 4th ed. 1984.

Muschel, L. 'Blood groups, disease and selection.' *Bacteriological Rev.*, 30, 2 (1966): 427–41.

Race, R. R., and Sanger, R. *Blood Groups in Man.* Oxford, England: Blackwell Scientific, 1975.

Sheppard, P. M. 'Blood groups and natural selection.' *Brit. Med. Bull.*, 15 (1959): 132–39.

Soulsby, E. H. L. 'Antigen-antibody reactions in helminth infections.' *Adv. Immunol.*, 2 (1962): 265–308.

Wyman, L. C., and Boyd, W. C. 'Blood group determinations of pre-historic American Indians.' *Amer. Anthropol.*, 39 (1937): 583–92.

——. 'Human blood groups and anthropology.' *Amer. Anthropol.*, 37 (1935): 181.

Blood types and lectins

D'Adamo, P. 'Gut ecosystems II: Lectins and other mitogens.' *Townsend Ltr. for Doctors*, 1991.

Freed, D. L. F. 'Dietary lectins and disease.' *Food Allergy and*

Intolerance, 1987: 375–400.

———. 'Lectins.' *British Med*. J., 290 (1985): 585–86.

Helm, R., and Froese, A. 'Binding of receptors for IgE by various lectins.' *Int. Arch. Allergy Appl. Immunology*, 65 (1981): 81–84.

Nachbar, M. S., et al. 'Lectins in the U.S. diet: Isolation and characterizatio of a lectin from the tomato (*Lycopersicon esculentum*).' *J. Biol. Chem.*, 255 (1980): 2056–61.

Nachbar, M. S., et al. 'Lectins in the U.S. diet: A survey of lectins in commonly consumed foods and a review of the literature.' *Amer. J. Clin. Nut.*, 33 (1980): 233845.

Norn, S., et al. 'Intrinsic asthma and bacterial histamine release via lectin effect.' *Agents and Action*, 12, 2/3 (1983).

Sharon, N., and Halina, L. 'The biochemistry of plant lectins (phyto-hemaglutinins A).' *Ann. Rev. Biochem.*, 42 (1973): 541–74.

———. 'Lectins: Cell agglutinating and sugar-specific proteins.' *Science*, 177 (1972): 949–59.

Schechter, Y. 'Bound lectins that mimic insulin produce persistent insulin-like effects.' *Endrorinology*, 113 (1983): 1921–26.

Triadou, N., and Audron, E. 'Interaction of the brush border hydrolases of the human small intestine with lectins.' *Digestion*, 27 (1983): 1–7.

Uhlendruck, G., et al. 'Love to lectins: Personal history and priority hysterics.' *Lectins and Glycoconjugates in Oncology*. New York: Springer-Verlag, date.

Uimer, S. J., et al. 'Stimulation of colony formation and growth factor production of human lymphocytes by wheat germ lectin.' *Immunology*, 47 (1982): 551–56.

Wagner, H., et al. 'Immunostimulant action of polysaccharides (he⁺ero-glycans) from higher plants.' *Arzneimittelforschung* 34 (1984): 659–61 (German abstract in English).

Waxdal, M. J. 'Isolation, characterization and biological activities of five mitogens from pokeweed.' *Biochemistry*, 13 (1974): 3671–75.

Zafrini, D., et al. 'Inhibitory activity of cranberry juice on adherence of type 1 and type P fimbriated *E. coli* to eucaryotic cells.' *Antimicrobial Agents and Chemoltherapy*, 33 (1989): 92–98.

The Lectins: Properties, Functions and Applications in Biology and Medicine. New York: Harcourt Brace Jovanovich/Academic Press, 1986.

Disease associations with blood type

Addi, G. J. 'Blood groups in acute rheumatism.' *Scottish Med. J.*, 4 (1959): 547.

Aird, I., et al. 'Blood groups in relation to peptic ulceration and carcinoma of the breast, colon, brochus and rectum.' *Brit. Med. J.*, 1954: 315–42.

Allan, T. M., and Dawson, A. A. 'ABO blood groups and ischemic heart disease in men.' *Brit. Heart J.*, 30 (1968): 377–82.

Billington, B. P. 'Note on the distribution of ABO blood groups in bronchiectasis nd portal cirrhosis.' *Australian Ann. Med.*, 5 (1956): 20–22.

'Blood groups and the intestine' (editorial). *Lancet*, 7475 (Dec. 3, 1996).

Buchanan, J. A., and Higley, E. T. 'The relationship of blood groups to disease.' *Brit. J. Exper. Pathol.*, 2 (1921): 247–53.

Buckwalter, et al. 'ABO blood groups and disease.' *JAMA*, 1956: 1210–4.

Camps, E. E., and Dodd, B. E. 'Frequencies of secretors and non-secretors of ABH group substances among 1000 alcoholic patients.' *Brit. Med. J.*, 4 (1969): 457–59.

——. 'Increase in the incidence of non-secretors of ABH blood group substances among alcoholic patients.' *Brit. Med. J.* 1 (1967): 30–31.

D'Adamo, P. 'Blood types and diseases, a review.' Clinical rounds presentation, Bastyr University 1982.

——. 'Combination naturopathic treatment of primary biliary cirrhosis.' *J. Naturopathic Med.* 4. 1 (1993): 24–25.

——, and Zampieron, E. 'Does ABO bias in natural immunity imply an innate difference in T-cell response?' *J. Naturopathic Med.*, 2 (1991): 11–17.

'Blood groups and susceptibility to disease: A review.' *Brit. J. Prev. Soc. Med.*, 11 (1957): 107–25.

Fraser Roberts, J. A. 'Some associations between blood types and disease.' *Brit. Med. Bull.*, 15 (1959): 129–33.

Harris, R., et al. 'Vaccine virus and human blood group A substance.' *Acta Genetica*, 13 (1963): 44–57.

Havlik, R., et al. 'Blood groups and coronary heart disease' (letter). *Lancet*, Aug. 2, 1969: 269–70.

Hein, O. H., et al. 'Alcohol consumption, Lewis phenotypes, and the risk of ischemic heart disease.' *Lancet*, Feb. 13, 1993: 392–96.

'An insight is gained on how ulcers develop.' *The New York Times*, Dec. 17, 1993.

Koskins, L. C., et al. 'Degradation of blood group antigens in human colon ecosystems.' *J. Clin. Invest.* 57 (1976): 63–73.

Langman, M. J. S. et al. 'ABO and Lewis blood groups and serum cholesterol.' *Lancet*, Sept. 20, 1969: 607–9.

Lim, W., et al. 'Association of secretor status and rheumatic fever in 106 families.' *Amer. J. Epidemiology*, 82 (1965): 103–11.

McConnell, R. B., et al. 'Blood groups in diabetes mellitis.' *Brit. Med. J.*, 1 (1956): 772–76.

McDuffie and Hart. 'The Behaviour in the Coombs test of anti-A and Anti-B produced by immunization with various blood group specific substances and by heterospecific pregnancy.' *J. Immunology*, 77 (1956): 61–71.

Martin, N. G., et al. 'Do the MN and JK systems influence environmental variability in serum lipid levels?' *Clinical Genetics*, 24 (1983): 1–14.

Myrianthopolous, N. C., et al. 'Relation of blood groups and secretor factor to amyotrophic lateral sclerosis.' *Amer. J. Human Genetics*, 19 (1967): 607–16.

'O! My aching stomach!' Witby *Republican*, Dec. 12, 1993.

Ratner, et al. 'ABO group uropathogens and urinary tract infection.' *Amer. J. Med. Sci.*, 292 (1986): 84–92.

Roath, S., et al. 'Transient acquired blood group B antigen associated with diverticular bowel disease.' *Acta Haematologica*, 77 (1987): 188–90.

Springer, G. F. 'Relation of blood group active plant substances to human blood groups.' *Acta Haem.*, 20 (1958): 147–55.

——, and Horton, R. E. 'Erythrocyte sensitization by blood group specific bacterial antigens.' *J. Gen. Physio.*, 47 (1964): 1229–49.

Struthers, D. 'ABO groups of infants and children dying in the west of Scotland (1949–51).' *Brit. J. Soc. Prev. Med.*, 5 (1951): 223–28.

Young, V. M., Gillem, H. G., and Akeroyd, J. H. 'Sensitization of infant red cells by bacterial polysaccharides of *E. coli* during enteritis.' *J. Ped.*, 60 (1962): 172–76.

Blood types and cancer

Aird, I., et al. 'ABO blood groups and cancer of the esophagus, cancer of the pancreas and pituitary adenoma.' *Brit. Med. J.*, 1 (1960): 1163–66.

Aird, E., et al. 'Blood groups in relationship to peptic ulceration, and carcinoma of the colon, rectum, breast and bronchus.' *Brit. Med. J.*, 2 (1954): 315–21.

Aird, E., et al. 'Relationship between ABO group and cancer of the stomach.' *Brit. Med. J.*, 1 (1954): 799–801.

Bazeed, M. A., et al. 'Effect of lectins on KK-47 bladder cancer cell line.' *Urology*, 32, 2 (1988): 133–35.

Boland, C. R. 'Searching for the face of cancer.' *J. Clin. Gastroenterology*, 10, 6 (1988): 599–604.

Brooks, S. A. 'Predictive value of lectin binding on breast cancer recurrence and survival.' *Lancet*, May 9, 1987: 1054–56.

——, and Leathem, A. J. C. 'Prediction of lymph node involvement in breast cancer by detection of altered glycosylation in the primary tumour.' *Lancet*, 8759, 338 (1991): 71–74.

Cameron, c., et al. 'Acquisition of a B-like antigen by red blood cells.' *Brit. Med.* J. July 11, 1959: 29–34.

D'Adamo, P. 'Possible alteration of ABO blood group observed in non-Hodgkin's lymphoma.' *J. Naturopath. Med.* 1 (1990): 39–43.

Dahiya, R., et al. 'ABH blood group antigen expression, synthesis and degradation in human colonic adenocarcinoma cell lines.' *Cancer Res.*, 49, 16 (1989): 4550–56.

Dahiya, R., et al. 'ABH blood group antigen synthesis in human colonic adenocarcinoma cell lines' (meeting abstract). *Proc. Ann. Mtg. Amer. Assoc. Cancer Res.*, 30 (1989): A1405.

Davis, D. L., et al. 'Medical hypothesis: Xenoestrogens as preventable causes of breast cancer.' *Environ. Health Persp.*, 101, 5, (1993): 372–777.

Feinmesser, R., et al. 'Lectin binding characteristics of laryngeal cancer.' *Otolaryngeal Head Neck Surgery*, 100, 3 (1989): 207–9.

Fenlon, S., et al. '*Helix popatia* and *Ulex europeus* lectin binding in human breast carcinoma.' *J. Pathology*, 152 (1987): 169–76.

Kvist, E., et al. 'Relationship between blood groups and tumours of the upper urinary tract.' *Scand. J. Urol. Nephrol.*, 22, 4 (1988): 289–91.

Langkilde, N. C., et al. 'Binding of wheat and peanut lectins to human transitional cell carcinoma.' *Cancer*, 64, 4 (1989): 849–53.

Lemon, H. 'Clinical and experimental aspects of anti-mammary carcinogenic activity of estriol.' *Front. Hormone Res.*, 5 (1978): 155–73.

——. 'Pathophysiological considerations in the treatment of menopausal patients with estrogens: The role of estriol in the prevention of mammary carcinoma.' *Acta Endocrin. Supp.*, 233 (1980): 17–27.

Marth, C., and Daxenbichiler, G. 'Peanut agaglutinin inhibits proliferation of cultured breast cancer cells.' *Oncology*, 45 (1988): 47–50.

Morecki, S., et al. 'Removal of breast cancer cells by soybean agglutinin in experimental model for purging human marrow.' *Canc. Res.*, 48 (1988): 4573–77.

Motzer, R. J., et al. 'Blood group related antigens in human germ cell tumours.' *Cancer Res.*, 48 18 (1988): 5342–47.

Murata, K., et al. 'Expression of blood group related antigens ABH, Lewis a, Lewis b, Lewis x, Lewis y, Ca19–9 and CSLEX1 in early cancer, intestinal metaplasia and uninvolved mucosa of the stomach.' *Amer. J. Clin. Path.*, 98 (1992): 67–75.

Osborne, R. H., and DeGeorge, F. V. 'ABO blood groups and

neoplastic disease of the ovary.' *Amer. J. Human Genetics*, 15 (1963): 380–88.

Renton, P. H., et al. 'Red cells of all four ABO blood groups in a case of leukemia.' *Brit. Med. J.*, Feb. 2, 1962: 294–97.

Roberts, T. E., et al. 'Blood groups and lung cancer' (letter). *Brit. J. Cancer*, 58, 2 (1988): 278.

Romodadnov, S. A., et al. 'Efficacy of chemo and immunochemistry in neuro-oncological patients with different ABO system blood group.' *ZH-Vopr-Neirkhiir Im Nn Burdenko*, 53/1, 17–20 (1989).

Stachura, J., et al. 'Blood group antigens in the distribution of pancreatic cancer.' *Folia Histochem. Cytobiol.*, 27, 1 (1989): 49–55.

Springer, G., et al. 'Blood group MN antigens and precursors in normal and malignant human breast glandular tissue.' *J. Nat. Cancer Instit.*, 54, 2 (1975): 335–39.

Springer, G., et al. 'T/Tn antigen vaccine is effective and safe in preventing recurrence of advanced breast cancer.' *Cancer Detection and Prevention* (in press, 1993).

Tryggvadottir, L., et al. 'Familial and sporadic breast cancer cases in Iceland: A comparison related to ABO blood groups and risk of bi-lateral breast cancer.' *Inter. J. Cancer*, 42, 4 (1988): 499–501.

Tzingounis, V. A., et al. 'Estriol in the management of menopause.' *JAMA*, 329, 16 (1978): 1638.

Wolf, G. T., et al. 'A9 and ABH antigen expression predicts outcome in head and neck cancer.' *Proc. Ann. Mtg. Amer. Assoc. Cancer Res.*, 30 (1989): A902.

Appendix H
Survey: Be a Part of the Blood Type Revolution

THE BLOOD TYPE REVOLUTION continues for all those who make the Blood Type Diet a part of their life. I am continuing to research the special conditions that the Blood Type Diets address, as well as the particular ancestries that seem linked to certain blood types and conditions.

I am very eager for your input. After you have followed the Blood Type Diet for at least three months or more, I welcome a report of what happened to you. I am also interested in hearing about adaptations you have made in menus and recipes that may be of use to others.

Your involvement in this work is an important contribution to the lives and health of others. Thank you for joining the revolution!

Part I: Background

Age ＿＿

Sex ＿＿ M ＿＿ ＿＿ F

Blood Type ＿＿ O ＿＿ A ＿＿ B ＿＿ AB

If you know your subgroup, include the information here:

Rhesus Group ＿＿ Rh+ ＿＿ Rh−

Secretor Status ＿＿ secretor ＿＿ no-secretor

MN Blood Group ＿＿ MM ＿＿ MN ＿＿ NN

Family Blood Type Tree
If you can find out the following blood types, it will enhance your understanding of the significance of your blood type

FATHER'S SIDE

your grandfather ____
your grandmother ____
your father ____

MOTHER'S SIDE

your grandfather ____
your grandmother ____
your mother ____

FATHER'S SIDE

your grandfather ____
your grandmother ____
your father ____

MOTHER'S SIDE

your grandfather ____
your grandmother ____
your mother ____

you ____
your children ____ ____

your spouse ____
____ ____ ____

Your father's ancestry: _____

Your spouse's father's ancestry: _____

Your mother's ancestry: _____

Your spouse's mother's ancestry: _____

Are there particular illnesses or diseases that run in your or your spouse's family? Yes ____ No ____
If yes, please elaborate.

Part II: Your Personal History
Do you have current medical conditions for which you are receiving treatment? Yes ____ No ____
If yes, please elaborate.

Do you have past medical conditions for which you have received treatment? Yes ____ No ____
If yes, please elaborate.

Have you ever had surgery? Yes ____ No ____
If yes, please elaborate.

Are you now or have you ever been on medications? Yes ____
No ____
If yes, please elaborate.

Would you consider yourself: ____ overweight
____ average ____ underweight

What is your profession? _____

Would you consider it ____ high stress ____ medium
stress ____ low stress

Would you consider yourself:
____ an exceptionally heavy exerciser
____ a regular exerciser
____ a light exerciser
____ no exercise to speak of

If you exercise regularly, what kinds of exercise do you enjoy?

What is your typical diet? List the foods you commonly eat.

Have you ever tried a special diet programme? If so, what was the
programme and why did you start it? What were the results?

Part III: Your Experience with
the Blood Type Diet

Why did you decide to try the Blood Type Diet? Give as much
detail as you can. For example, did you or a member of your
family have a medical condition that you thought could be
helped? Did you decide after reading the book that this approach

offered the opportunity to take further control of the choices you make now that will affect you in the future?

How long have you been on the Blood Type Diet? ____

What were the most difficult adjustments for you to make?

Have you also followed the exercise recommendations? If so, what have you noticed about your stress level and general state of conditioning? If you changed radically from the exercise style you were used to (i.e., from running to yoga), describe that change. Do you feel it's worked for you, or not?

What has been your overall experience with the Blood Type Diet?

(If applicable) Have your partner and your children also tried the Blood Type Diet? If so, what has been their experience?

Have you come up with any terrific recipes or alternative foods that have made the Blood Type Diet work for you? If possible, please enclose them.

Have you found good ways to balance the needs of family members with different blood types? Please share them.

Do you have any final observations about the value of the Blood Type Diet that you would like to share? I welcome comments that might lead me to further clarify my work.

THE POWER OF READING

(optional)
Name: _____
Address: _____
City: _____   State: _____   Zip _____
Phone: _____

Would you be willing to be contacted about your experiences with the Blood Type Diet? Yes _____ No _____

Would you like to be put on a mailing list to receive updated information on blood type research and therapies?
Yes _____ No _____

Are you interested in receiving information on ordering home blood-testing kits? Yes _____ No _____

Thank you!

Return this survey to:
   PETER D'ADAMO, N.D.
   Survey
   P.O. Box 2106
   Norwalk, CT 06852–2106
   U.S.A.